TIDAL WAVES
The Moments of Me

B. AMBER STARK

NFB
Buffalo, New York

Printed in the United States of America

Tidal Waves: The Moments of Me/ Stark 1st Edition

ISBN: 978-1-953610-41-6

    1. Mental health awareness> books
    2. Motivational self-help> books
    3. Personal transformation self-help
    4. Mental health guide
    5. Memoir

NFB
NFB Publishing/Amelia Press
119 Dorchester Road
Buffalo, New York 14213

For more information visit Nfbpublishing.com

Dedicated to:

My mom, dad and sisters for your undying support, help and advice on both the good days and the bad days. For never giving up on me and for having faith in me.

My nieces, for giving me a new purpose in life and the grounds to maintain my stability.

My extended family, especially my Aunt Mary Jane and my Aunt Rosemary, for your ongoing support.

My loyal companions, for the joy and happiness you bring to me on a daily basis.

Thank you to all who have stuck by my side through this journey which is what helps carry me through.

Table of Contents

"No one saves us but ourselves
No one can and no one may
We ourselves must walk the path"
-Buddha

PREFACE

We all go a little mad sometimes. I think that is something we can all agree on. And by madness, I mean experiencing an unstable mind. How people deal with their madness and overcome it is what matters most. I don't think it matters how it starts so much, but how someone carries on after such an experience. I, myself, have fallen victim to the short fuses of my own mind. To be precise, I had mental health episodes in 2013, 2015 and 2016. *TIDAL WAVES: The Moments of Me* is about the three mental breaks I had. I chose this title because my episodes all came out of nowhere and hit me like a tidal wave and they were all moments of my life. Moments that don't define me as a person per se, but that helped me grow as a person.

Throughout the book I try to paint mental pictures of a reality that I thought existed. Delving into the thoughts and ideals that drove my madness. The format of my story was difficult to piece together considering the fact that a lot of things I remembered came to me in fragments and not necessarily a sequenced timeline. The sequence of my first episode was probably the easiest of the three for me to recall. This is likely due to the fact that I talked about my experiences of my first episode immediately following my hospital stay. However, the second and third episodes are scribed in no particular order. The sequence in which they happened was not 100% clear for me because I did not talk about these experiences afterwards. However, I did try to make my thoughts as coherent as possible. Throughout the book I mention that certain stimuli "spoke to me." I want to clarify that I did not hear voices. Rather, stimuli triggered certain thoughts in my mind that made me think they were directives or signals from outside forces.

TIDAL WAVES: The Moments of Me is a book of six sections. The first section is titled ICEBREAKER which is about my first episode. I decided to name it ICEBREAKER because it seems to have been the icebreaker to my severe unstable moments. The second section is named MANIC MIND which is about my second episode. My second episode was a manic break. MANIC MIND includes Facebook posts I shared during that time. I presented the posts the way I wrote them when I was manic. These posts are free of editing because I wanted to capture the authenticity of the posts with how they were originally written in my manic state. The third section is named HOSTAGE. I decided to call it HOSTAGE because I felt like a hostage in my own home during the course of my third episode. The fourth section is named RECOVERY: THE GOOD FIGHT and is broken down into three sections. The first section in RECOVERY: THE GOOD FIGHT is the First Stretch of Recovery following my first episode. The second section is the Second Stretch of Recovery following my second episode. And the third section is the Third Stretch of Recovery following my third episode. I still consider myself in my third stretch of recovery to this day. Since this section is about my recovery, I chose the title RECOVERY: THE GOOD FIGHT because I feel that a stable mind and a fulfilling life are worth fighting for. The fifth section is called LIFEBUOYS. Lifebuoys are defined by Wikipedia as "life-saving buoys thrown to people in the water to provide buoyancy. They usually have a connected line allowing them to be pulled in." I chose to call this section LIFE-BUOYS because it refers to my family and how they were affected by my experiences over the years. To me, my family members are my lifebuoys and have helped me to battle through and have buoyed me up out of the darkness in my life. They continue to do so every day. I want to acknowledge them, especially my sister Ava, for sharing their thoughts and allowing me to incorporate their side of the story into this book. The sixth and final section of this book is called CALM WATERS. I decided to call it this because I have a sense of serenity and peace now. The tidal waves seem to have calmed down. I feel I am definitely in a better place as if I'm swimming in calm waters. This section includes things I have learned and advice I share that will hopefully help others in need that may be struggling in any way.

If it wasn't for my family and the road to recovery I have taken, my mind would still be spiraling out of control. With certain tools and supports, I can confidently say that there is a way out of the madness. That there is an avenue which, with the right methods, can lead one back to a stable mind and a fulfilling life. Which leads me to the main purpose of this book. Not only did writing this book help me personally. But I also wrote it with the hopes of helping others by giving them an insight into a reality they may share with me on some levels. I think writing about my experiences has helped me come to terms with this small portion of who I am. And doing this has helped me recover more successfully. Putting my paranoid thoughts to paper and reading them gave me the opportunity to see how I was driven by irrationality during my episodes. In turn, I am now able to identify irrational thoughts that seep in and talk through them and not feed into them. So, to anyone who may be suffering, I urge you to put pen to paper and release it. It was one of the best therapies for me. I hope my story shines light on the fact that there is a way out of a dark tunnel.

"Storms are hauntingly beautiful
  Their calm can be preciously petrifying
  Life is a storm
  It is hauntingly beautiful
  It is preciously petrifying"
-b. amber stark

PROLOGUE

THE SUMMER OF 2013, I was a stable-minded young woman. I held a job as an administrative assistant in a school, lived in an apartment with my boyfriend of eight years, owned two dogs who I cared for dearly, received a Master's degree in psychology, and was living a life that one would consider, for the lack of a better word, normal. I spent my free time away from work hanging out with family and friends. In my alone time I often found myself blaring music and dancing around the house. Like many individuals in their mid-twenties, I lived a relatively care-free life. I never gave much thought to or realized the importance of one's mental health. And I never really felt as if I was emotionally or mentally unstable. But unexpectedly, in the fall of 2013, that all changed....

"Rip the sanity from my mind the way the wind rips the flame from a fire on a windy night

Freeze my emotions leaving me stuck with fear in the face with no hope for a way out in sight

Blind me with delusions and cripple me with paranoia causing me to lose all my might

Bleeding anxiety that suffocates me and captures me from the light

This life is like being coiled inside the spindles of a spider's web, stiffened from defense and no way to fight"

-b. amber stark

Section I
ICEBREAKER

Paranoia has set in full force. I started living a life of analyzing and dissecting everything around me on a daily basis. Trying to put together the pieces of a puzzle that in reality did not exist. For example, while driving I would spot someone in my rearview mirror, considering them suspicious and I would get the notion that they were following me. Out to get me for some reason. After weeks of experiencing these thought processes, things started to spiral out of control. To the point that I was starting to think that my own boyfriend, Paul, and my other good friend (who was our roommate) were now plotting against me. I started getting suspicious about things around the house. I would experience odd smells, and began thinking that my roommate was planting some chemicals in the house that were creating the toxic odors I was smelling. He worked in a bio lab and I was convinced he was bringing them home. The boys were also set on the idea of getting a gun license. Now initially this did not faze me, but as time went on and paranoia set in, I started to think otherwise. I started to get suspicious. They often watched the T.V. show "The Walking Dead." Their obsession with "The Walking Dead" and their desire to get a gun license began to creep me out. I was now convinced that they were picking up ideas from the show. After some time, I started to think that the boys were out to get my family and me. I'm from a predominantly Irish family and they were both Italian. With the way my mind was working I began to associate my suspicions regarding the boys' interests to the mafia.

One day we were in the car pulling out of the driveway and my roommate noticed the man passing by on the sidewalk and mentioned how he looked like the father of one of our friends. He chuckled about it. I was in full freak out mode at that point - on the inside. Sitting silently in the back seat, I started creating scenarios in my mind. Wondering why he had said that. I thought that he must have said it because it really was my friend's father. And now I was under the impression that "my friend's father" was also there to help organize the mafia's attack on my family and South Buffalo. South Buffalo, the town we lived in, is known for its Irish Heritage. So, I began to believe it was a target for the Italian Mafia too. Aside from being freaked out about the boys and my thoughts about the Italian Mafia, I also felt people were following me and that my phone was being tapped. I remember I started to notice that whenever I would unlock/lock my car, the number of beeps that sounded would change. Sometimes it would beep once or twice, other times it would beep three times. This made me paranoid into thinking that my car had a tracking device and that I was being traced whenever I would enter or leave my car. I believed the tracking device would also track wherever I went so that my location was disclosed at all times. My paranoia had reached a high point. I truly believed what I was thinking and was becoming a prisoner of my own irrational thoughts.

But even though I was freaked out, I tried to remain calm and keep living my life.

One particular day I returned home from work and greeted my boyfriend. As he greeted me back, he made an off-hand comment about finally submitting his application to get his gun license. Since I was suspicious about all the scenarios spiraling in my mind over the past weeks, I was overcome with extreme fear when my boyfriend made the off-hand comment. It was the culmination of all the fears and paranoia that had been building up and I finally reached my breaking point. So, when my boyfriend got in the shower, I seized the opportunity and grabbed my dogs and ran out of the house. I didn't even close any doors. I was beyond terrified. I hopped into the car and started driving towards my parents' house. I started crying. Suddenly I changed my mind and made a quick turn to instead go to the cemetery to visit the gravesite of my great aunt, who had recently passed. I was headed down the main road to the cemetery when I became suspicious of the man in the red car behind me. I thought to myself that I needed to lose him, so I quickly made a right hand turn down a side street and sped to the stop sign. At this point I was extremely terrified. Therefore, instead of going left to the cemetery, I made another right hand turn to head back to my parents' house. As I turned right, I noticed the man in the red car approaching the stop sign on the street parallel to the one I just came from. I was still under the impression he was following me. Feeling desperate and scared, I laid on my gas blowing through four stop signs, making a right hand turn and continuing to my parents' house. I pulled into the driveway and jumped out of the car leaving it running with my two dogs inside. I ran into the house to find my dad. I was crying hysterically and told my dad I didn't trust the boys anymore and I was terrified. I felt that something bad was going to happen. My family did their best to calm me down, but I think it became clear to them that something was not right with me and they grew concerned. Later that night my family and I sat down in the living room and had a discussion. They said they wanted to take me to the hospital, Erie Community Medical Center (ECMC) to be evaluated. At first, I was reluctant to go. But after some convincing I told my family I would go the next day.

TUESDAY, OCTOBER 22, 2013

My parents and I arrived at ECMC and we were sitting in the waiting room. I found two individual men in the waiting room suspicious and I was under the impression that they were a part of "the team" that was against my family. However, they were not sitting together. One man was standing in the corner of the waiting room on his cell phone. I felt he was communicating with outside forces on his team regarding their plot against my family and me. The other man would not stop staring at me. He resembled a female friend of mine who was also Italian, like my boyfriend and my roommate. So, I thought he too was against my family, part of the Italian mafia. I was so terrified that I discreetly had to snap a picture of him with my cell phone in case I needed it as evidence if anything were to happen. I finally was called back to the first-floor private waiting room. I was somewhat comfortable as I was the only one in there at the time. First, I met with a nurse and I explained to her how I had been feeling paranoid and scared. I gave her some history of the events leading up to my episode. I lost all control and broke down into tears. I explained to her that in the recent past I had experienced two great losses - the death of my childhood dog and the death of my great aunt. They were both very important to me and I considered them two of my best friends. So, losing them both in such a short period of time really took its toll on me. These significant events were so traumatic and may have been what contributed to the unstable mindset and paranoia I had begun to experience. I can't help thinking that I may have been better off if only I had taken my mother's advice from years prior: learn to control your emotions, don't let your emotions control you. Instead, after these two losses I had let my emotions get the best of me and chose poor outlets to self-medicate: drinking and smoking pot.

After meeting with the nurse, I was sent back to the private waiting room. My family was not allowed back there, so I was alone. The hospital had "The Big Bang Theory" and "Family Guy" on the T.V. Both shows felt like they were applicable to me, to the people in my life, and just seemed as if they were about my life. That was another symptom I was experiencing. The shows "spoke to me" and were giving me insights on my own life. I felt I related so much to what was happening in the episodes that I thought they were actually about me and were purposely played in the waiting room specifically for me to see. I found this to be peculiar but was not necessarily scared about it. I was more so enlightened by each episode.

I finally had the chance to meet with the doctor who also listened to my story and the symptoms I was experiencing. He went in to meet with my family separately. After meeting with my family, the doctor determined it was best I stay the night. The hospital had two main areas for patients experiencing mental health symptoms. We came to know them as the "loud floor" and the "quiet floor." From my understanding, the quiet floor was designated for patients experiencing a lesser degree of mental distress and therefore had less distractions and disruptions. The loud floor was designated for patients with more severe symptoms and who required a longer stay. The hospital didn't have a room opened on the quiet floor so they had me stay in a small room off of the private waiting room for the night. The doctor felt that the alternative floor would be too loud for me at the time and would exacerbate my symptoms. So, they arranged for me to spend the night in the private waiting room until I was able to be moved to an open room on the quiet floor. The bed I was placed in for the night was in a little room. There was also another bed in the room assigned to another patient. We did not interact. She pretty much slept the whole time. With everything going on in my mind, I was skeptical about being in a room with a stranger. I just laid in the bed, under the covers with my mind racing. Across from the doorway was a window to another room with a closed door. I noticed a woman in there. She appeared irate and kept pounding on the window. She kept screaming over and over that she needed her medicine. I laid there terrified, thinking about what would happen if she broke out of the room. I was afraid she would attack me. I tossed and turned all night, with wide eyes, not sure what to expect.

WEDNESDAY, OCTOBER 23, 2013

The following morning, I was transferred to the quiet floor. The first night on the quiet floor I was in one of the common areas watching T.V. by myself. One of the other patients on the floor approached me and started talking to me. I recall her being really good with remembering dates of historic events. She carried on with conversations about historic events as well as other random topics. Every once in a while, the nurse would come by to make sure she wasn't bothering me. I reassured the nurse I was not bothered and actually enjoyed the other patient's company. Some of her comments even made me laugh. She was one of the sweetest people I've ever met and actually made me feel more comfortable and not so alone. Shortly after our conversation we both headed to our own rooms for the night. I remember one of the nurses brought me a case with contact solution so I could take out my contacts. However, being paranoid, I thought that the solution was tainted with chemicals, so I refrained from taking them out.

I made it through the first night on the quiet floor and anxiously waited for my family to arrive for visiting hours the following day. It actually happened to be my mother's birthday that day. When my family arrived, we hung out in the visiting room and played the game "Apples to Apples." I was making connections with the cards from the game. Associating the cards that my family members would play with a sign or message that I believed they were trying to give me. These signs/messages were positive in nature. I felt comforted and content. The fearful thoughts seemed to have subsided with my family there by my side. We all enjoyed each other's company with a lot of laughs from the game. We sang "Happy Birthday" and had cake. Before I knew it visiting hours had expired. It was such a wonderful visit. A change in pace from where my mind had been. It was hard to watch them leave. I wanted to go with them. I wasn't looking forward to being alone again in a strange place, with irrational thoughts to top it off. But it was time for my family to leave. So, we said our goodbyes until visiting hours the next day.

Friday, October 25, 2013

I hung out with a few of the other patients in the common area. There was a movie playing which made me think of my family and the situation I was experiencing. Although I am not sure of the title of the movie, there were two specific parts of the movie that "spoke to me." First, a young boy was left in charge of watching his younger brother and failed to do so. I remember the father yelling at the older brother because something bad had happened to the younger brother. I do not remember exactly what it was because as the movie was playing, I became distracted talking to another patient at the table; a woman who resembled, and who I actually thought was, Mary-Louise Parker from the T.V. show "Weeds." However, I do remember there being a negative situation in the movie where the young boy was abducted or possessed by demons/negative energy through his bedroom window. My mind had me thinking that the movie was telling me that this was something that happened to me in the past. The older brother represented my older sister, Carlie, and the younger brother represented me. I thought that it was something traumatic I may have repressed in my mind and had just now come to the realization from watching the movie. I felt as if the negative energy I encompassed from the traumatic event was being brought back to life and it was one of the reasons why I was in the hospital. The second part of the movie had to do with a character in the movie named Ellen that was friends with the father. Being a huge fan of Ellen Degeneres, this had me thinking that my father actually had a personal friendship with Ellen Degeneres. The significance of my father's "personal relationship" to Ellen meant that she was going to help me get out of the hospital. At first, I couldn't believe my father never told me they were friends back in the day since I've always been a big fan of hers. But then I realized it was all part of the "game" and he was not allowed to tell me. At this point it was as if life was a game of balancing positive and negative energy. I felt that if I played my cards right and was able to balance out the positive and negative energy in a ratio of at least 3:1, respectively, then things would be peaceful and everyone would be safe from all negative energy.

Shortly after the movie, a doctor came and met with me in my room. He asked me if the movie I watched "spoke to me." I did not go into detail, but I did say it was applicable to me and my life to a certain extent. He also asked me to describe how I was feeling. I told him that I felt energy - some things came off as positive energy, whereas others came off as negative energy. From that point forward, this concept played a major factor in how I thought about everything and anything, and also in how I behaved. After a few more questions the doctor left the room.

My friend Nick, who I had known since college and who was currently in his residency at the time at ECMC on another floor, stopped by on his break to visit me. My family had reached out to him to let him know I was admitted to ECMC. We sat at the table talking as I explained to him how I was feeling. Dinner, which consisted of a pasta dish with red sauce, was served as we continued talking. I took a bite of my dinner and found that it tasted funny. I refused to eat it as I thought it was poisoned with chemicals. He tried to reassure me that it was not. But that seemed to be one of the symptoms I was having where I experienced odd tastes and smells. Soon enough it was time for Nick to leave.

While hanging out and waiting for my family, I remember a man in the common area looked at me and very excitedly said, "It looks like someone is going to fly on an airplane to London tomorrow morning." I immediately thought he was talking about me. On the inside I was ecstatic because I thought this meant I was getting out of the hospital. I truly believed he meant that my sister, Carlie, and I were going to go to London to be on a talk show. And to add to my excitement, I saw a helicopter on the launch pad at the hospital for emergency flights and I thought that was where we were going to have to go to get on our "private flight."

Shortly after this, visiting hours approached and my family arrived. They spoke with the doctor who told them that I had said the movie was "talking to me." This was an indication that my symptoms were getting worse. Therefore, he felt it was best if I remained at the hospital. My family was nervous about this as it would mean I would have to move to the loud floor since my allotted time on the quiet floor was up. To my knowledge, the quiet floor was reserved only for patients who stay for a maximum of 2-3 days. After 2-3 days, patients either get discharged or get transferred to the loud floor depending on their status. I finished visiting with my family that night, and the following morning I was transitioned to my new room on the loud floor.

After my family received the news that I would be staying at the hospital for the foreseeable future, they requested a meeting with the doctors at the hospital. They were looking for more concrete answers about my status and were still scared and confused about what was going on with me. After some back and forth and persistence on their part, they were granted a meeting. They were placed in a conference room at a table across from doctors who seemed unaccustomed to this type of thing - to someone's family being so involved and asking so many questions. This was sad because it highlighted the fact that so many people who suffer with mental health issues in this country don't necessarily have the support system that I am so lucky to have. Don't have loved ones being involved, demanding answers, and advocating for them. Sadly, for many, the mental health ward becomes a revolving door. In and out, in and out again. So, when my family requested that meeting, it was clear that the doctors were trying to keep their patience with them and to answer their questions. At one point when my family expressed confusion about what was happening, it seemed as if all the doctors and specialists in the room exchanged glances, as if they had already reached a foregone conclusion, and that my family had not quite caught up yet as to what exactly was going on. One of the doctors looked at my mom and said "listen, I understand that it can be hard. A 'first break' can be hard. To watch your child, who up until this point appeared healthy and happy, go through this and to accept that they're sick is difficult." "First break?" What did they mean by that? What was a "break" and by "first" did they mean that there might be more to come? Would this be a persistent life-long issue rather than a little hiccup with a quick fix? My family told me it was at that point that my mom broke down. She buried her face in her hands and let out a cry. I believe that might've been the moment it sank in for her. That I was really, really sick. And that the road ahead would probably not be an easy one for me.

Saturday, October 26, 2013 - The start of my 2-week hospital stay on the loud floor

My first night on the loud floor there was a Buffalo Sabres game on T.V. in the smaller common area. I decided to venture in and watch the game. There were two male patients in there at the time. We began talking by discussing the reason why each of us were at ECMC. Tim, one of the male patients, was also giving me tips about being there since it wasn't his first time. One thing he told me was that if anyone was chasing me or bothering me to go to my room because patients are not allowed in other patient's rooms. He said the nurses will tackle down any patient who tries to enter another patient's room. This concerned me a little bit. But I appreciated his tips and immediately connected with him and felt as if he was positive energy. We continued to talk about hockey. I noticed he was sporting a Chicago Blackhawks Kane 88 hoodie, which I took as a sign that he was there to help me. Tim and I were both fans of Kane because he was an All-Star hockey player that was born and raised in Buffalo, NY. As we were watching the Sabres game, we discussed how it would be cool if one day Kane could play for his hometown. As the game concluded it was time to head to our rooms for the night.

At this point paranoia was getting intense and I was starting to hear things. I was lying in my bed that night working on a word find. I heard someone enter the floor from my end of the hallway, which was farthest from the nurses' station. As the person walked down the hall and back, it sounded like they were dragging their feet. I also heard clock ticking noises and pictured an evil clown carrying a clock. The ticking was creepy as it sounded like a ticking time-bomb, which I imagined the clown was holding as it staggered down the hall. I was too afraid to get up and check. This was all negative energy to me. It seemed like every 20 minutes I would hear the creaking of the door opening and closing, which was followed by the so-called evil clown staggering back and forth down the hallway with the ticking time-bomb. This scared me and increased my anxiety more and more each time. Needless to say, I had a hard time sleeping that night.

The next morning, I was awakened by a nurse who came in to draw my blood. She told me she did not know what the bloodwork was for but was doing as the doctor ordered. Half asleep still, I did not make anything of this at the time. After the bloodwork I met with other patients at the nurses' station for meds, weigh-ins and to get blood pressure checked. Afterward we all proceeded to the meal room for breakfast.

Following breakfast, the pacing would begin. Some patients on the floor would spend most of the day pacing, including myself. Other patients would spend most of the day sleeping. Certain patients and staff members would feed me either negative energy or positive energy. I felt that my purpose was to help offset the patients who had negative energy in order to maintain stability, positivity and peace. I thought that if I was able to prevent patients from creating negative energy, it would increase positivity and peace. Positivity and peace, not just on the loud floor and at the hospital, but also around the world. With this mindset, I thought one patient, Marcus, was the head of all negative energy. Therefore, it was important for me to interact with him and neutralize his negative energy in order to prevent bad things from happening.

One particular day, Marcus and I were walking the hallway and were just talking about whatever came to mind. He would often bust out into raps that I thought he made up but I was never able to understand what he was saying. However, I saw it as his way of exorcising his demons in a positive way so I reassured him that his songs were creative. At one point we stopped in the hallway in front of a mural that was painted on the wall. It was a beautiful picture of a sunset over a crashing wave. Marcus told me however, that if I looked at it from a different perspective, it looked like a big fire and like something was burning. This creeped me out and reassured me that he was in fact the head of negative energy. I began to think that his view of the picture as a fire was allowing negative energy on the floor. I gave him a small nod and told him I prefer to perceive it as the beautiful sunset. That it's the same concept as whether or not you choose to see the glass as half empty or half full; whether you choose a positive mindset and outlook or a negative one.

It was almost time for visiting hours. I anxiously waited for my family to arrive. At this point, my paranoia seemed to have grown worse than it was when I initially arrived. I continued to pace around the floor, going from one common area to the other. The small room represented positive energy whereas the bigger room represented negative energy. This information is important as it plays a huge role in what I perceived to be the purpose of why Tim, one of the first patients I met, and I were at the hospital. In my mind it was our purpose to prevent negative energy from taking over the smaller, already positive room and to constantly create enough positive energy to take over the "negative energy" room. I would always see the word "LOVE" printed in chalk on the cage over the window in the negative room. I was under the impression that Tim was the one who would keep writing it on the window day after day, as it would get cleaned off every morning. I thought "LOVE" printed in big letters had spread positive vibes and helped create positive mindsets to anyone that entered the negative room.

As I waited for my family, I noticed that the pitcher of water that was set out for patients and guests had a pink tinge to it. The pitcher also had a number on it each day. I thought it was the room number of the different patients on the floor, especially since one day it had my room number on it. I believed that the water was mixed with the blood from the patient whose room number was on the pitcher. I believed that was the reason why the nurse had to draw my blood the first morning that I was on the loud floor. My family arrived and I warned them not to drink the water. I was also suspicious of a medication they were giving me and described the pill to my family. I asked my sister, Natalie, to go home and Google it so I knew what I was taking. They asked how I was doing. My sister, Carlie, told me that if I was not honest about how I was feeling a lot of people that I love would be seriously hurt. I told them I was doing okay and I was happy to see them. At the time, it was how I was feeling. I felt okay with them there. But deep down I was terrified to tell the truth about all the paranoid thoughts in my mind when I was alone at the hospital. To me they were not thoughts, they were reality. I felt if I told them what I was thinking when they were not there, terrorists would kill my family and innocent civilians. In that specific moment, I thought they were going to bomb the hospital and kill everyone in it if I talked about anything. Even though I was having these thoughts, I kept my composure because I was grateful for my family being there and felt okay in the moment. We continued with small talk until visiting hours were over.

That night I was sitting in my bed, juggling between doing word searches and attempting to read a book. I felt that these were two ways to increase positive energy. As I was working on a word search, a light caught the corner of my eye from the window. I looked up and noticed a helicopter flying toward my room. Paranoid out of my mind, I thought the helicopter was headed toward my window and I dove from my bed to the ground. My heart was racing. As I dove, I perceived the helicopter to be making a swift turn, flying away from my window. I imagined the helicopter was hijacked and that two people were wrestling with each other in the helicopter. One person, the hijacker, was trying to fly it into the hospital to kill me and the others in the hospital. The other person, the pilot, was fighting to steer the helicopter away from the building. I was terrified. Once again, I had trouble sleeping. I went down to the nurses' station and asked if I could talk with one of the nurses. They initially told me they had work to do and weren't able to. But I told them that the nurse on the quiet floor had told me that if I ever needed to talk to anyone, I could always talk to one of the nurses. At that point, one of the nurses on duty sat and talked with me in the common area. After talking I felt a little better and went back to my room to attempt to sleep. Being terrified, I felt the need to increase the positive energy in my room. Another way I felt I could increase positive energy was by praying. I laid in bed and started reciting prayers I learned growing up, including the "Hail Mary" and the "Lord's Prayer." I sat in bed reciting these prayers over and over. I would juggle between writing down the words and doodling pictures of Holy Mary and crosses in the blank spaces of my word search book. Also, it was a must that I used the color purple because at that moment in time, to me, purple encompassed the most positive power.

On a side note, another thing that I would do was wear a beanie hat at all times. I felt I had a glow around my head similar to a halo and believed that wearing a beanie would disguise it from being noticed by any of the evil staff and patients. I would also apply lotion all over me, including my hair. I believed that doing this had similar camouflaging effects as wearing the hat did. This was a tip I picked up from Tim. Tim barely had any hair and would apply lotion to his head. However, it was not something he told me to do, it's just something I saw him doing one night. That was one way I communicated with others. They did not necessarily have to tell me to do something, but just seeing it done made me think that it was something I needed to do too. Something I needed to do in order to protect myself, which trickled out to protecting my family. As time went on, the hospital grew cold and I would cover myself with a brown blanket that my parents had brought me, which I believed had protective powers. I believed the cold atmosphere was a good thing and that it meant good spirits were surrounding me.

The next morning, patients lined up for our daily routine of meds, weigh-ins, and blood pressure readings. I was feeling pretty tense as we entered the room for breakfast. Brandi, another patient on the floor, along with Tim, noticed that I seemed off, as I was fully covered by my brown blanket from head to toe. This was due to the fact that I was terrified from all my irrational thoughts, not because I was cold. I felt protected by the blanket. So, they came over to console me as I had my head covered by my blanket. I was refusing to make eye contact with anyone. Barely even with them even though I befriended them when I initially arrived. One of the reasons I felt comfortable with Brandi and Tim was because of their names. They both share names with two of my friends. I took this as another sign that they were sent to the hospital to help me. That morning, I did not have an appetite and did not eat much. I headed back to my room to do a handstand to help exorcise my demons and rid myself of the negativity I was feeling. After a few handstands and some yoga poses, I found myself in the bigger common area collecting pages from magazines that "spoke to me." Spoke to me in a sense that I felt the pictures, words, and articles were positive energy. I stored these items in my room. At that point I was invited to go to one of the groups with a few other patients. We went to another floor where we all created our own shirts. We were all given a plain white t-shirt and were presented with a bunch of sharpies. We were making tie-dye shirts by drawing with different colored sharpies and then painting the image with alcohol to make the colors bleed like a tie-dye design. My images consisted of a peace sign, happy face, yin yang, and four swirly designs. One swirly design was made of blue and red which represented the Buffalo Bills, the second one consisted of blue and gold for the Buffalo Sabres, the third one was purple and white which represented Niagara University, and the last one was gold and brown which represented St. Bonaventure University. The Buffalo Bills and the Buffalo Sabres were my hometown sports teams. Niagara University and St. Bonaventure University were where my sisters and I attended college. I chose these four different color combinations as I felt all four were composed of good energy and helped fight off the negative energy in the world. This shirt became magical to me as it encompassed positive energy in several ways. I wore this shirt throughout the rest of my stay.

Shortly after our group session, my father arrived for afternoon visiting hours. He greeted me with a hug and a kiss. Since I was still tired due to not getting much sleep from the night before, I leaned on my father's shoulder and took a snooze while he was there. The comfort of having him there made me feel content. I took a quick cat nap and woke up after about 20 minutes. When I woke up, my dad began to talk about the buildings that could be viewed from the visiting room window. There were three specific buildings, but I can only recall the one being a church. After our conversation, I noticed another patient, Darryl, in the room watching a soccer game. He looked nervous as the team he was cheering for needed another goal to win. Now, to me sports teams either provided positive vibes or negative vibes to the world. Specific details of a team would determine which type of energy the team contributed to the world. For example, color combination was one main aspect that determined whether a team was "good" or "bad." However, one color could manifest in different ways depending on the situation or context. In other words, the color red could denote positivity for one team or situation, but negativity for another team or situation, depending on other variables involved. Aspects other than color combinations that played a role in how I viewed a team included location, school, fans, and numbers (whether it be the score or a player's jersey number). Whatever the aspects may have been in determining a "good team," it was always important for the favored team with the positive energy to win. For example, the Buffalo Bills, Buffalo Sabres, and Chicago Blackhawks were teams that carried positive energy. So, it was always important for them to win because if they lost, bad things would happen. Things such as natural disasters and terrorist attacks. In this situation, this particular patient gave me good vibes, and the team he was cheering for had green jerseys which to me meant positivity. Therefore, I felt it was important for his team to win. As the game grew intense and time was running out, the team he was rooting for pulled it off and scored a goal. Both of us were very excited and gave each other a high five. As the game concluded, he left the room satisfied. As visiting hours ended, my dad said goodbye and told me he would be back up to see me for the evening visiting hours.

After my father left, I went back to my room. I stood in front of the window and peered out into the distance at the buildings my dad had mentioned earlier. I had my blanket covering my head. As I stood there someone came to my room and said in a strange voice, "Barbara-ann, Barbara-ann." This creeped me out for two reasons. One reason being that is not how to say my name. The other reason being that the person speaking sounded like a gremlin. It made my hair stand on end. I froze. They continued reciting what they thought was my name. They even grabbed my shoulder and tried to get me to turn around. I continued to ignore them thinking it was extremely important I remained calm, still and quiet. I was afraid if I turned around, I was going to be shot in the face. Finally, they left my room. I continued to look at the buildings, making note of the distance between each one. I thought I was going to need to know this because there was going to be a flood. I figured my dad pointed the buildings out to me because he was giving me hints on how to survive. When this so-called flood would hit, I would use my wooden bed as a boat and would have to row from one building to the next in a specific pattern in order to help people survive. The final destination would be the church. As I was looking out the window, I also noticed a platform directly outside the window about four stories below my room. There were suspicious looking items on the platform that were orange. I had it in my mind that these items were bombs. It was up to me to make sure I did the right thing in order to prevent them from blowing up. I also believed my sister Ava's boyfriend, Brian, was going to be the one to defuse them.

After looking out my window I decided I needed to venture into Brandi's room which was adjacent to mine. It was connected through the bathroom that we shared. I knew that we weren't allowed to be in other patients' rooms, but the nurses were not able to see me since I was entering through the bathroom. I felt really out of it and scared, and wanted to talk to Brandi. So, I entered her room and walked to her bed, but she was sleeping. I noticed that her roommate Shakira had a felt cardboard cross displayed on her dresser. The cross signified a very powerful tool to me. The idea of walking around the floor with the cross in an effort to spread positivity crossed my mind. I wanted to ask Shakira if I could borrow her cross but she was not in the room at the time.

That night my boyfriend, Paul, came for evening visiting hours with my father. I was only allowed so many visitors at a time, so everybody would take turns coming to see me. My boyfriend looked really worried and upset which I knew had to do with the fact that I was in the hospital. But still, I was thrilled to see him. We hung out and watched T.V. in the smaller common room. There was a Fallsview Casino commercial that came on T.V. that suddenly got me thinking that people were trying to break us up. It was a commercial where a boyfriend and girlfriend were out to eat and the servers from the restaurant brought out a cake with a sparkler as a candle and sang a breakup song. The song went, "Breaking up, breaking up, breaking up is hard to do. She met you and liked your face but now she really needs her space. You're done, you're done. You were two and now you're one." Again, this had me thinking there may be evil forces trying to break us up. This was obviously just an irrational thought in my mind and thankfully he was very supportive at the time. Even with these thoughts clouding my mind, I was grateful to have him there and believed that we were not going to let the negativity break us apart.

After my visitors left, I found myself walking around the floor with my blanket around me. Not necessarily because I was cold, but still feeling that it protected me. Similar to the book, "The Hunger Games," I thought my family would bring me things to benefit me during my stay. Things that would protect me from the evil energy on the floor. This included items such as the brown blanket, word searches and a pair of slippers that had an owl face on them. I met Tim in the small common area (or what I considered the positive common area), where we were working on our word searches. Every time I worked on a word search I would use a specific color crayon. The color crayon I would use depended on the energy I was feeling based on the thoughts I was having. And it was important to use the right color as it would create the greatest amount of positive energy possible. After a little while, Tim left to go to the bigger common area. A bunch of patients were playing charades so he went to join them. I thought it was important for me to continue working on the word searches while Tim went to "trump" the negative energy in the bigger common area. I saw this as teamwork in radiating positive vibes.

I returned to my room for the night where I began to surround myself with all the positive magazine pictures and articles I had collected. I was also under the impression that the "bloody pitcher water," which had my room number on it that night, was fed to the other patients, which meant they were more prone to attack me. Kind of in the sense that drinking the water would cause them to want more of my blood, like a vampire. To prevent them from coming into my room, I placed my owl slippers at the edge of my bed. The edge of my bed hung out past the wall and was the only part of my bed visible from the hallway. In my mind, this tactic would scare off any attackers. I felt the slippers had protective powers and that the owl eyes would intimidate anyone trying to intrude and attack me. Also, to me the owl slippers symbolized the goddess, Athena, who is the goddess of war, strategy and wisdom, and who is often accompanied by an owl.

I sat in my bed with all the magazine clippings surrounding me. I believed that putting the positive images, sayings and articles around me helped to increase the positive energy in my room. Therefore, if any "negative beings" entered my room they would feel these vibes and be brought down and be less likely to attack me. I was feeling pretty anxious and scared, trying to figure out ways to create more positive vibes. I remember lying in my bed with the covers over my head. At one point, a nurse came in and found me lying on the bed, surrounded by all of the magazine clippings.

Another thing that disturbed me was the fact that I saw little bugs flying around my head. I was under the impression that these bugs were video cameras and that I was being watched. So, I laid in bed swatting at and fighting off these bugs, which to this day I'm not even sure were real or just a hallucination. At the same time, I was anxiously shuffling between trying to read books, and complete word search and crossword puzzles. But unfortunately, it became too hard to even do these activities that had previously brought me a sense of calm because now they too had begun "speaking to me." These activities now made my paranoia and fear even worse. It got to the point that the clues in the crossword puzzles seemed to tell a story, a story with negative connotations. To clarify, completing the puzzles was one way of creating positive vibes. However, sometimes the different word searches and clues from the crossword puzzles would have me paranoid and creating scenarios in my mind. I did not just see them as words that shared a common ground or phrases that were clues to the puzzle. But as words and phrases that were telling a story or sending me a message. And at times, the story or message manifested in a frightening way. I also remember trying to read the book, "When a Tree Grows in Brooklyn," but slammed the book shut after a couple of pages on two different occasions. The thoughts from reading and trying to complete the puzzles were fear-ridden. Therefore, I again began to pray. I would continuously recite the "Hail Mary" and the "Lord's Prayer," and again write them down on the pages of the word search and crossword puzzle books that screamed negativity to me.

The next day following breakfast I joined a group activity where we had the opportunity to color felt images. I found the same type of felt cross that Shakira had displayed in her room. I quickly grabbed the cross and colored it purple and yellow. I believed that this cross was an important tool to have for the remainder of my stay. After the craft session, I had another group activity which consisted of a ditto worksheet. The ditto consisted of healthy eating and necessary exercise needed to maintain a stable mind. Group ended and I was greeted by my father and cousin, Kirstin, for afternoon visiting hours. My cousin asked how I felt. I told her I was okay. But then I started crying and told her I just wanted to get out of the hospital and be back home. She said she understood and reassured me that this was only temporary.

After visiting hours ended, I found myself pacing with Marcus. We were discussing random topics as I focused on keeping him calm. With a suspicious grin, he said he wanted me to come with him to California to sell bottles of water with someone he referred to as "Uncle." I thought that this was code for him wanting me to go with him to be a sex slave. I was afraid to say no because I was not sure how he would react. I thought he would possibly hurt me. Just to appease him, I laughed and said, "okay." Marcus wanted me to talk to "Uncle," who I later was convinced was actually the rapper DMX, on the phone. So, we went to the phone, where he called "Uncle" and he put me on the line with him. The guy on the other end of the phone said, "So you want to come and sell water bottles with us?" Marcus walked away and I panicked. I played along and told "Uncle" that I would help. But feeling freaked out on the inside, I dropped the phone, leaving it hanging off the hook, and walked away.

My mom and sisters arrived with dinner. My sister Natalie made me pasta with red sauce, green peppers and chicken. I was too afraid to eat the food from the hospital unless it was pre-packaged. Therefore, my family would bring me something every day during visiting hours. For this, I was extremely grateful.

After visiting hours, patients were allowed to go to the recreation room on the fourth floor. This included patients that were staying in the other wing of the loud floor. There were all sorts of activities to engage in, including foosball, Play Station, Wii and listening to music. There was also a treadmill, as well as a small gymnasium with athletic equipment. There was even an outside porch area for those who wanted to get some fresh air. When I got onto the elevator there were two patients from the other wing standing there. The female patient chuckled and said to me, "Oh I know why you're here." I was confused by her comment and found it peculiar. The other patient was a male who to me resembled Noah from the Bible story "Noah and the Ark." He was a thin man with medium length white hair and a short white beard. He was phenomenal at playing foosball. It was magical and he would always play when we would venture to the fourth floor. Of course, to me this was one of his ways of radiating positivity. The fact that he looked like Noah from the Bible further validated to me that there was going to be a flood as I had suspected earlier. However, the twist on the story was that my bed was going to be the boat and I was the one that would have to travel through treacherous waters and reach the church to save everyone. After connecting ideas in my mind, it dawned on me that this was what the female patient from the elevator must have meant when she said, "I know why you're here." She somehow knew I was there to save everyone from a flood. After watching "Noah" play foosball, I went to check out the gymnasium. There was another patient from the other wing shooting around with a basketball. He was wearing a purple shirt. I saw him as good energy, as I saw the color purple as being loyal. I joined him in shooting around as we cheered each other on to sink the baskets we were attempting. Of course, making a 3-point shot was the most powerful in terms of creating positive energy. Soon after this, recreation hours concluded and all patients went back to their respective wings for the remainder of the night.

On Saturday, families arrived for visiting hours and my mom, dad and sisters came to see me. I was still under the impression that my blanket had protective powers. The nurse came to my room to notify me that they were there to visit. I proceeded to slowly walk down the hallway completely covered by the blanket from head to toe, like a ghost. The only thing showing were my feet. I held the blanket in a way where I could see the floor by my feet. I would pay attention to any shadows reflecting on the floor which let me know if something or someone was in the way of my path. I greeted my family all covered up with the blanket because I was having a bad day and I was terrified. I sat in the chair in between my mom and my sister, Natalie. I curled up in a ball on the chair, still completely covered by the blanket. They kept gently trying to get me to come out from under the blanket. But I thought they had guns to their heads and would be shot dead if I did. I must have refused to take my medicine that day as they were trying to give me some. I was still afraid to take it but then started to think if I didn't, they would be shot in the head. Therefore, after refusing for about ten minutes and coming to the conclusion that they would be shot if I didn't, I reached just my hand out from under the blanket and took my medicine as I remained covered. They kept asking me what was wrong and if I was cold. I lied and said nothing was wrong and yes, I was just cold. In my mind I felt like I was being tested. I was afraid to say what I really thought was going on. I thought terrorists had guns to their heads, trying to get me to come out to witness them being brutally shot and killed. I was envisioning it. I was terrified and scared for my family. After their continuous attempts to convince me to come out, I finally took the blanket off to find that everything was alright. It was just them and no terrorists with guns. Obviously, they noticed I was not doing okay and comforted me until they had to leave.

There was a patient that stayed in the room behind the wall with the sunset mural. I thought he was evil and possessed by the devil. He was not very nice to me. I remember he was a scrawny man with round glasses. I thought he would transmit his negative vibes through the wall to the bigger common area which was adjacent to his room. When we would go to the recreation floor, he would always run on the treadmill. I thought that was his way of spreading his negative vibes. Therefore, I would go in the gym which was adjacent to where the treadmill was on the other side of the wall. I would position myself in front of the section of the wall in the gym where he would be running on the other side. I would kick a soccer ball as hard as I could repeatedly at that section of the wall. I had it in my mind that the power from the ball hitting the wall would prevent him from running at his best and break down his ability to spread his negative vibes.

I was hanging out in the bigger common area alone one night when Marcus came into the room. I remember him smelling like alcohol which was not surprising as there were visitors who would sneak cigarettes and alcohol in for certain patients. Apparently, Marcus was one of them. I actually recall one of the patients smoking in their room. But this night Marcus tried to make out with me. He kept asking me for a kiss. Now since he was drunk, I felt it took away from his ability to spread negative energy. Therefore, I had the upper hand in the sense of spreading good vibes. I remember telling him that the doctors and nurses could see us. There was a globe-like fixture that was like a mirror on the ceiling by the window and I convinced him it was a hidden camera. Partially because I really thought it was one. After explaining that to him, he finally gave up on the whole kissing idea.

Throughout my stay I had no concept of time or any idea about what was going on in the outside world. But it was the end of October and close to Halloween. I never made the connection. So, when Tim showed me a Halloween decoration his nephew had made for him, I freaked out. I thought it was a bad omen at first and tried to rip it apart. Tim was quick with his reaction of protecting the decoration from getting destroyed. After thinking about it for a while though, I thought Tim was actually showing me because he was trying to tell me that jack-o-lanterns were a way to fight off the evil patients and staff members. That explained why he reacted as if he was trying to protect it. I remember one night I could not sleep so I went to the small common area. I brought a paper bag and I drew a jack-o-lantern on one side. I shimmied the chairs into the corner forming a box with the wall, so I could fit between them. I crouched down in the corner, between the chairs and held the bag in front of me with the jack-o-lantern side facing out. I thought the two staff members on shift that night were aliens and would be scared off by the powers of the jack-o-lantern. They came to check on me and could not find me at first. They came into the room, looked around and left with a concerned look on their faces. Minutes later they returned and finally realized I was hiding behind the jack-o-lantern bag, between the two chairs in the corner. They ordered me to come out. They were not happy with me to begin with because I was not supposed to be in the common area. I refused to leave the common area. I was not being aggressive. I was just standing stiff and would not exit the room. At this point, they started to try and physically direct me to my room. This terrified me to the point that I actually peed my pants. After a little fighting, I convinced them to let me watch T.V. in the common room. I ran down to my room to change and grabbed my pillow, blanket, and sheet. I had a plan in my mind that I was going to sleep in the common area since I was too afraid to sleep in my own room. After I returned to the common area, I positioned the chairs side by side and made a little bed to lie down in. I set my sheet inside with my pillow and after I hopped in, I covered up with my blanket. There was a camera on the ceiling right outside the common area that would capture activity in the hallway. However, I was under the impression that the camera was focused in on me through the window separating the hallway and the common room. I was content with this, as I thought the camera would capture if anything were to happen to me and alert hospital security. Eventually, I fell asleep.

As I mentioned before, I felt that certain sports teams possessed positive vibes, notably the Chicago Blackhawks NHL team. Buffalo native Patrick Kane, who was one of the Blackhawks' star players, was a key person in creating positive energy. One particular night, the Blackhawks were playing a game at the United Center in Chicago. I thought the Blackhawks needed to win, otherwise the United Center would blow up, killing everyone inside. Therefore, when I was alone in the smaller common room during game time, I was meditating in a sense. Kane is #88. In my mind I would create positive vibes for the Blackhawks by meditating, walking eight floor tiles in one direction and eight floor tiles back. I did this back and forth while stating in my head, "with Kane, we are able." I paced along the tiles a total of eight times. I was content in my mind thinking that this would help guide the Blackhawks to a victory and save people from dying.

One night, most patients were asleep. It seemed as if the tactics that Tim and I used to create positive vibes were working. This particular night, Tim, Brandi, Darryl and I were hanging out in the bigger common area with nothing but positive vibes to spread. We were playing the card game Uno. Each color in the deck signified a different strength of positivity. During this game, yellow was the strongest. As the game progressed it reached a point where we kept flipping yellow cards. It seemed endless. And to me it signified nothing but positive vibes. And we were also in the "negative" common area. So, I thought we had met our goal and had overcome the evil energy on the floor and had conquered the negative energy around us. Thus, the positive energy trickled out into the outside world and contributed to peace around the world. After our game, we were flipping through a coloring book. Tim stopped at a picture of the Rescue Rangers. We both looked at each other and laughed and it felt as if we were thinking the same thing. It was like we had gotten over the peak of our mission of radiating positivity - on the floor and in the world as a whole. As if we were the "Rescue Rangers." The bigger negative common area was now overflowing with love and good vibes.

As it was getting late, everyone started to return to their rooms to sleep. However, I did not leave right away. I sat in the bigger common area at the table because I thought it was finally that time that I'd been waiting for - the moment I was going to get out of the hospital. Not only that, but the singer, Pink, and the comedian/T.V. show host, Ellen Degeneres, would be the ones to come and help me get out of the hospital. After all, "my mission" was now complete. So, I sat and waited patiently, coloring to pass the time. After about fifteen minutes I noticed a shadow in the doorway of the common area. I was overcome with excitement because I knew it was them. Followed by the shadow was a security guard who just peeked his head in, glanced at me, and walked out. Seeing the security guard had me thinking he was making sure the coast was clear to bring Pink and Ellen in to see me. After about five minutes I was curious that nobody showed up. So, I decided to get up and see where the security guard went. I exited the room into the hall and looked toward the nurses' station at the end of the hall. All I saw were two nurses and the security guard. I was pretty bummed out. However, at that point, I convinced myself maybe it wasn't the night Pink and Ellen were going to help me get out. I told myself, "Patience is a virtue," and they will arrive when the moment is right. It was my duty to maintain the positive vibes on the floor until they arrived. I headed back to my room and called it a night.

The next day in group I colored a picture of a bedroom. While lying in bed later that evening, I made a connection between the image I had colored and my room at the hospital. If I held the image up a certain way, items in the picture lined up with things in my room. For example, when I held up the picture in a specific way, the bed in the picture lined up with the bed in my room. There were flowerpots set up in two different spots in the picture. There were light switches in my room exactly where the two flowerpots were located in the picture. There was one next to my bed and one next to the entryway to my room. So, I thought I had to flip the switches by the bed in a certain combination in order to unlock the gate that covered the window in my room. I thought that this would provide me with an escape route from the hospital. I spent quite some time fiddling with the light switches, trying to unlock the gated window. I thought that if I could figure out the right combination of flicking the switches, I could escape. I was under the impression that my family was going to save me by picking me up with a helicopter. I was going to escape by jumping out of the window and onto the helicopter. Every once in a while, you would hear "code red" announced over the intercom in the hospital. I thought this meant someone else had escaped, or tried to. I kept trying different combinations of flicking the light switch by my bed on and off, followed by pacing back and forth in groups of eight, and then trying to open the window gate. Needless to say, I had no luck getting the window gate open. The nurse came in, and found me standing on my bed. He asked what I was doing. Concerned that I was still awake, he told me to get down and to go to bed. I am sure the random flickering of the lights coming from my room had alerted the nurses.

The next day Tim told me he was going to be getting discharged from the hospital that coming Friday. I asked him for advice on how I could get out of the hospital too. He told me that one of the doctors comes in every Tuesday morning and that he was the one I needed to talk to. However, I had just missed the doctor, as this was on a Wednesday. So, I had to wait a whole week before I could talk to the doctor. That past Tuesday, I remembered seeing this particular doctor walk by as I was in the room they called "the purple room." It was called the purple room because it had lavender walls, a purple recliner and a purple rug. They had brought me in there because I was refusing my oral medication because I was paranoid it was going to harm me. Without understanding my fears, the nurses told me I needed to take the oral medication. Otherwise, they would have to administer the medication with a shot. I was then afraid of the idea of getting a shot because I thought it was going to kill me in a matter of minutes after taking it. I had three nurses around me continuing to convince me to take my medication. While this was going on, I noticed a doctor walk by the purple room. In hindsight, I realized he was the doctor Tim was telling me I needed to talk to in order to get out of the hospital. While the nurses continued to try to get me to take my medication with concerned looks on their faces, I eventually grew terrified that something bad was going to happen. To be specific, I thought a plane of terrorists was going to fly into the window of the purple room if I did not take my medicine. So, I agreed to take my oral medication. Aside from talking to the doctor, Tim also said to make sure to attend every group session that the hospital offered.

One day there were workers fixing the light fixtures in the ceiling of the main hallway in the wing I was staying in. However, at the time I believed they were actually defusing bombs that had been planted in the ceiling. I believed that the hospital was rigged with bombs and that people in the hospital, including myself, were being set up to die. But the positive vibes that Tim and I had emitted on the floor had helped to prevent the bombs from being detonated. Our tactics in creating positive vibes had helped outside forces gain control of the people threatening to detonate the bombs. After seeing what I thought were bombs in the ceiling get defused, I felt safer on the floor than I did originally.

A new male patient arrived. His name was Phil. Since Tim had left, Phil had basically taken over Tim's role in terms of being my partner in spreading positive energy. I thought Phil resembled members of my family, especially my father. I thought he was literally my dad's child with another woman, or maybe a long-lost cousin of mine. I truly thought he was a relative and I wanted to introduce him to my Aunt Teresa and my cousins, Tyler and Jamie, when they came to visit. However, Phil was sleeping when they came and I never had the chance to.

Tuesday morning, I made a point to wake up early and walk around until I found the doctor Tim had told me about. Luckily, I was able to find him and I told him I was ready to go home. He asked me if I was taking my medications. I told him yes and he said, "okay." That was the extent of our conversation. Needless to say, I was relieved and excited. By this time my medication had kicked in, my paranoia/fears had pretty much subsided and my mind was starting to stabilize again. The positive energy was at a greater level than the negative energy at this point in my mind. It was all about maintaining the positivity from that point on.

Tuesday night, recreation hour had arrived. Phil and I headed out to the patio deck to get some fresh air. When we got out there Shakira had the radio playing and was listening to music. I couldn't help but start dancing. At one point I decided to pull out my signature dance move, "The Worm." This was a great moment in my mind because Shakira and I were dancing together, spreading good vibes.

The remainder of my stay mostly consisted of different group sessions, as well as Phil and I hanging out. My paranoia subsided and my mindset seemed to be improving. My last night at the hospital finally arrived. Phil and I were hanging out in the big common area, where there were apples for our late-night snack. There were two left. At that point, Phil and I each grabbed an apple and took a bite. All I could think of was the creation story of Adam and Eve. I said to Phil, "This isn't like the forbidden fruit, is it?" He replied, "I hope not." We both chuckled and left the room. I felt lighter and more positive than I had in awhile.

The next day, I was finally released from the hospital. I was eager to get out of there as you could imagine. My parents arrived and we met with one of the discharge nurses. I remember she advised that I continue to take my medication. She told me that if I went off the medication, other people would be able to realize that something is not right. I said alright and agreed, signed some paperwork and I was on my way home.

This is where the journey of my recovery began. I spent the first few weeks after being released from the hospital at my parents' house, as they figured this was the best thing for me. My boyfriend would come and spend time with me there. The first few days being home and out of the hospital seemed to be alright for the most part. I wasn't experiencing paranoia or delusions. However, my anxiety had sky-rocketed and I was having panic attacks. This manifested in not only mental ways but also physical. I remember one of the first few days I was experiencing a lot of pain in my back. I asked my boyfriend if he could rub my back. I believed it was sore due to the anxiety I was feeling. I explained to my mom and boyfriend that it felt as if "angel wings" were growing out of my shoulder blades. It was painful. My boyfriend rubbed some stress relief lotion on my back for me. Followed up with some deep breathing, the attack dissipated.

When I came out of the hospital, I was set up with a chemical dependency counselor because I was an excessive pot smoker before I went into the hospital. I would meet with the chemical dependency counselor once a week. She would talk to me about several topics. Some topics included the importance of staying clean, what drugs do to my mind and body, how they could have contributed to my episode and how continuing to use pot increases the risk of another episode. She would also provide me with information regarding various workout classes in the area that would help aid in my recovery, such as Yoga and Zumba.

I was also set up with a mental health counselor, who I met with once every two weeks. My mental health counselor would take updates on how I was doing mentally and physically, how I was handling work once I went back, and gave me strategies and techniques to help combat my anxiety. I was set up with a psychiatrist who I met with monthly and who helped manage my medications.

About a month after being discharged from the hospital I moved back into my apartment with my boyfriend. Around this time, I was also given the opportunity to apply for a new job. This job was important to me as it was a job that enabled me to put my Master's Degree in Psychology to use. I tried my best to make the job work, but the levels of anxiety that I would experience on a daily basis hindered my ability to focus. I found aspects of the position to be overwhelming and unfortunately was not able to continue. It's like I was at the right place at the wrong time. I had no choice but to part ways and move on. Luckily, I had the option to go back to work at my previous job, once I got the clearance from my psychiatrist saying it was alright for me to return. After a few short months of being on a leave from work, I was cleared to return to work in February of 2014.

My recovery was pretty tough. I experienced depression and I was very sluggish. I slept a lot and just did not do too much in the beginning. But I continued to battle through and listen to what my counselors and psychiatrist would say. I was honest with them about the way I was feeling since I believed it was the only way for me to get the right and most effective treatment needed. And if I had a beer or two, I would tell my substance abuse counselor. But for the most part I stayed away from drugs and alcohol.

I continued with my recovery, attending counseling, meeting with my psychiatrist and taking my medications. After about a year, it was determined that I had made progress mentally. Around the same time, my boyfriend made the decision that he would be joining the military. Initially, when he told me he would be leaving I was upset and sad at the thought of not having him around. I regret to say that this kept me from being fully supportive of him at first. But after having conversations with him where he said that this was something that would benefit our future together, and that him being away would only be temporary, I became more receptive to the idea. And ultimately after realizing that this was something that was important to him and something that he really wanted to do, I supported him in the decision. When the time came for him to leave for training, I was left with the hope that this was something that would be good for us in the long-run.

While he was away at training, I remained optimistic and was overall happy. I had reached a point in my recovery where I had been maintaining mental stability. And in mid-May of 2015 I concluded my final counseling session. I was happy, as my progress was good news to share with my family and my boyfriend. I was especially excited to tell my boyfriend since he'd been gone at training for about four months at this point. While he was away, we managed to communicate and stay in contact through e-mails. He would often e-mail me about how much he missed me and how he wanted to move on to the next chapter in our relationship and get a house together once he returned. The e-mails I would receive from him would leave me feeling happy and hopeful for our future. However, when the time came to finally see him again, I was confused by his actions. I had traveled with his family to attend his graduation from military training. But he did not really seem happy to see me when I arrived. It was clear something was not right. The person I saw that day was not the same person I had been e-mailing and talking to over the past few months. And once we returned home to Buffalo after his graduation, it wasn't even a full four weeks before he suddenly left without warning one day and never returned.

To say I was blindsided is an understatement. I thought we were going to be together forever. He had led me to believe that, especially with what he said in his e-mails and during our phone calls while he was in training. When looking back and trying to make sense of things, I realize that in those weeks following the graduation, he had begun to act distant. I would go to work during the day and when I would return home he would not be there. I would call him to see where he was and he would be an hour away at his parents' house. He would tell me he was coming home but he wouldn't show up until later in the evening. He did this a number of times throughout the course of a week, where he would randomly leave without notice while I was at work. Looking back, I now realize he must have been slowly removing his belongings from our apartment and moving them to his parents' house while I was at work. However, this was not apparent to me at the time because he did leave some of his belongings behind. After about a week of this, one day I returned home from work to again find he wasn't there. I tried to call him several times. But this time he never answered my phone calls. He would not respond to my text messages either. With no warning, or explanation, my boyfriend of ten years had walked out of my life.

This left me confused and upset. I cried for a week. I would blare and sing to "Just One Reason" by Pink and "All I Want" by Kodaline. I would sing these songs until I could without crying. Confusingly though, my emotions at the time kept fluctuating between sad and happy. On one hand, I was completely devastated that my boyfriend had walked out on me. On the other hand, I was elated as a result of a hypomanic state that I was experiencing, which I did not realize at the time. Being in the hypomanic state made dealing with my boyfriend walking out easier. I definitely still felt upset but it was like the hypomania had numbed me to the full magnitude of the situation. I still felt sad and would cry, but no one really saw me upset because I was always alone when I expressed it. My family only saw me happy following him leaving and they found it to be odd and alarming. Even though I was confused about how the relationship ended so abruptly, I refused to let him take away the positive mentality and good feelings I had been experiencing due to the elated state I was in from the hypomania. So, I fought through the tears and tried to focus on the positive.

One good thing I had going for myself was a friendship I built with my colleague, Rhee, from work. To stay happy, I would occupy myself with caring for my dogs, spending time with my family and hanging out with Rhee. I looked to my family for support in regards to everything going on with my boyfriend at the time.

There were several red flags during this time that tipped my family off and made them begin to think that something just wasn't right. They were concerned about me. In addition to how they saw me react to my boyfriend leaving, I had also informed them that I'd e-mailed my superiors at work regarding a "grand idea" I had. I had e-mailed the board members of the school district I worked for, and suggested that teachers should display the Golden Rule, "treat others the way you would like to be treated," in classrooms for students to learn. My family thought that reaching out to the board members was a risky move. They were in fear of me losing my job. I would also post strange statuses on my Facebook page. The posts were usually rambling and hard to follow. And I would go off on a tangent and the posts would be lengthy. I got to the point where I was getting little sleep and my behavior was getting reckless. Another thing that alarmed my family was that I had a pair of bongos that I would often play while I was driving. They were starting to become concerned for my physical safety. And similar to my first episode, I was "feeling energy" again. But this time around, it started with positive vibes rather than negative vibes. These positive vibes were overwhelming and became a prominent element in what was to lie ahead. Unbeknownst to me, I was heading down the second hill of my mental rollercoaster. I was slipping into a manic episode.

"Hit me like a tidal wave
Holding me captive from clear thoughts
You stole my rationality
In a sea of mind-warping juggernauts"
-b. amber stark

Section II
MANIC MIND

"5:00 in the morning, so we meet again." Staying awake all night seemed to be the trend those days. Sleeping did not seem to be an option. I was running on about one to two hours of sleep a night. My mind was running wild. Rapid fire. Floating on cloud nine. I spent my days working followed up with some vino and pot. Yes, I got back into drinking...and smoking pot again. And I felt invincible. No sleep had my days bleeding together. Along with my thoughts bleeding out of my mind with positivity. I couldn't help but share with the world.

Not even my boyfriend of ten years walking out on me could break the intense vibes I was feeling. Alright, it did catch me totally off guard at first, considering all the love letters and plans of a future together that he had been putting in my head. Again, I spent the following days after he left repeatedly listening to "Just One Reason" by Pink and "All I Want" by Kodaline. Blaring them as loud as I could, singing as loud as I could, until I could conquer the tears with a sudden control. It wasn't about love. It was ultimately about respect. And clearly, he didn't respect me.

Facebook Post June 25, 2015:

im learning that its not really about love...its about RESPECT. In order for two people to work, there needs to be a rich mutual respect for one another. Without respect there can be no love. RESPECT ...and the LOVE will follow...and that's not just for two people that want to spend a life together...I feel it goes for WHOEVER you cross paths with in life...whatever happened to the golden rule: TREAT OTHERS THE WAY YOU WANT TO BE TREATED.

Facebook Post June 27, 2015:

"Right from the start you were a thief you stole my heart and I your willing victim. I let you see the parts of me that weren't all that pretty and with every touch you fixed them. Now you've been talking in your sleep, oh, oh. Things you never say to me, oh, oh. Tell me that you've had enough of our love, our love. Just give me a reason just a little bit's enough just a second we're not broken just bent and we can learn to love again. It's in the stars it's been written in the scars on our hearts. We're not broken just bent and we can learn to love again. I'm sorry I don't understand where all of this is coming from I thought that we were fine (oh, we had everything). Your head is running wild again my dear we still have everythin' and it's all in your mind (Yeah, but this is happenin') You've been having real bad dreams, oh, oh, you used to lie so close to me, oh, oh there's nothing more than empty sheets between our love, our love. Just give me a reason just a little bit's enough just a second we're not broken just bent and we can learn to love again."

- "Just Give Me A Reason" by Pink

These were the lyrics to the song "Just One Reason" by Pink and they were so relatable for me at the moment. And I was letting the positive notes of the music carry me on - "we're not broken just bent, and we can learn to love again." This song allowed the light back in after a brief darkness that I refused to let consume me.

Facebook Post July 3, 2015:

"We have one chance, one chance to get everything right, we have one chance one chance and if we're lucky we might. My friends my habits my family they mean so much to me."

-"One Chance" by Modest Mouse

Regardless of the fact that my boyfriend had walked out on me, I had my family there by my side. Supportive as always, especially when I needed them most. I also spent most of my time with my new friend, Rhee, and she felt like a soulmate. It was like we crossed paths through fate.

Rhee and I spent time exchanging stories over some vino, pot and cigarettes. We often stayed up late even on work nights. The one night we stayed up until sunrise, tapping into our creative spirits. I spent the early hours of that morning putting an idea I had in mind to paper. I had been pondering about healthy crutches vs. toxic crutches in life. And I seemed to be engaging in the latter. So, I drew a picture about it. In the picture the top states: Choose your crutch wisely. And from there the picture was split in half by a flower. One side of the stem had dead flowers whereas the other side of the stem had an image of healthy blossomed flowers. The side with the dead flowers had a caption that read "One will make you stuck." It had a drawing of a beat-up person with a sad face that had crutches made out of cigarettes with smoke streaming from them. There was a box of beer on the ground next to the person. The sky had clouds with rain and lightning bolts. This side of the picture represented the toxic crutches in life that keep you stuck and prevent you from getting ahead. The other side with the blossomed flowers had a caption that read "One will set you free." It had a drawing of a person with headphones listening to music, dancing underneath a clear sky and sunshine with a rainbow. There was a butterfly, flowers, a frog, and a set of bongos next to the person. This side of the picture depicted the healthy crutches in life that help you escape the lows and move up mountains to a better place.

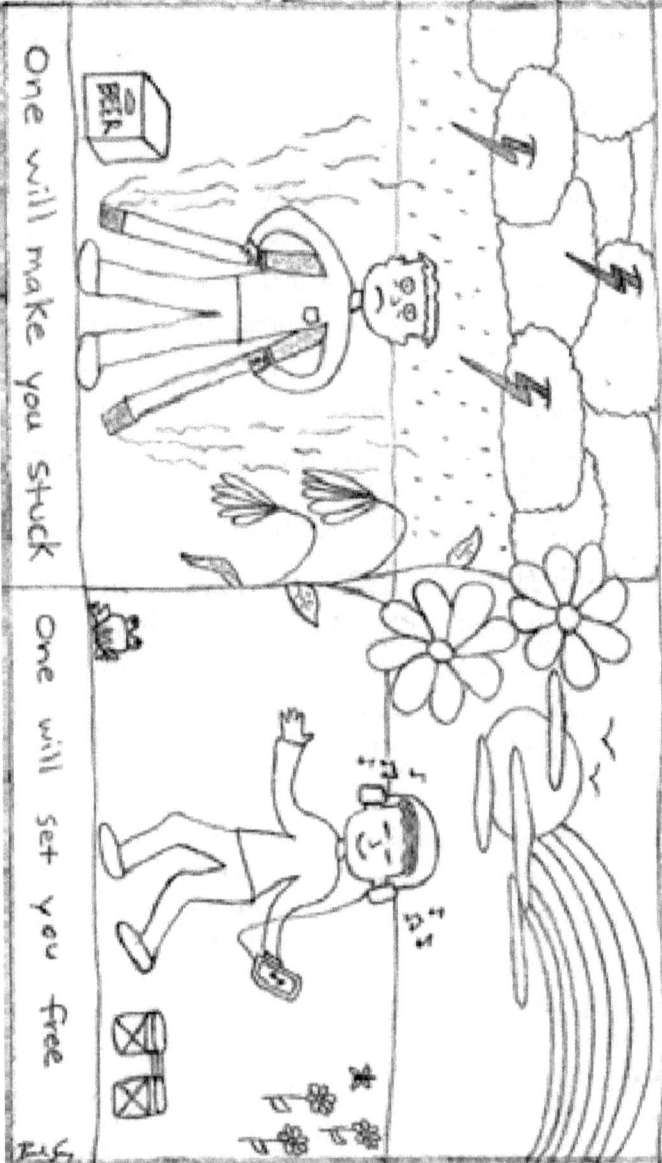

Music had become one of my biggest crutches. It carried me through my days. Whether it was helping me get over my recent breakup or helping me explore my feelings. And the influence of music was apparent in my daily Facebook posts, which were made up of song lyrics that resonated with me during that time.

Facebook Post July 4, 2015:

"So you can keep me inside the pocket of your ripped jeans. Holdin' me closer 'til our eyes meet. You won't ever be alone. Wait for me to come home. Loving can heal. Loving can mend your soul. And it's the only thing that I know (know). I swear it will get easier. Remember that with every piece of ya. And it's the only thing we take with us when we die."

-"Photograph" by Ed Sheeran

Facebook Post July 5, 2015:

"I never thought I'd see the day you didn't take my breath away but that day has come. I never thought there'd be a time your hand wasn't placed in mine but now you're gone. And I know better than that not now and I thought we could work it out. And maybe you will come around but you won't. So I'll let you go. Now that I know. That life won't lead you back to my door. Not long ago they said to me someday soon it set me free. I tell them that they're wrong and I believed in every word you said. You were just fucking with my head and stringing me along. But I know better than that now and I thought we could work it out. And maybe you will come around but you won't. So I'll let you go now that I know that life won't lead you back to my door."

-"Back To My Door" by John Higgins

Facebook Post July 8, 2015:

"To me you are more than just skin and bones. You are elegance and freedom and everything I know. So come on and baby, let your hair down. Let

me run my fingers through it. We can be ourselves now go ahead, be foolish. No one's on the clock now. Lying in this simple moment. You don't gotta worry now. Just let your hair down."

-"Let Your Hair Down" by Magic

I hadn't been single in ten years. The thought of someone not by my side at night was unsettling. Not having that someone to turn to when you need them. Not understanding why "all of a sudden" he chose to leave. Especially when things seemed so good. Especially when we had been contemplating our future together. And just ALL OF A SUDDEN, he is gone. But after a lot of thinking and musical outlets, I came to terms with it. Maybe not forever but for that moment. All the fears that he triggered within me; the fear of not having him around, the fear of being alone - I was being forced to overcome them. And I did it. And I felt free.

Facebook Post July 9, 2015:
Fight your fears, set yourself free.

Facebook Post July 11, 2015:
Rolling Stones at Ralph Wilson Stadium

On the night of July 11, 2015, I went to the Rolling Stones concert at Ralph Wilson Stadium. It was quite the party. Family. Beer. Pot. And Dancing. A lot of dancing. I was overcome by the music and refused to leave my seat for not even a second to visit the restrooms. I was feeling elated and energized, and overcome by the music and the joy of being at the show. Since I didn't want to risk leaving and risk missing out on any of the concert, I ended up losing control and peeing my pants.

Facebook Post July 12, 2015:
Would you pee your pants for a once in a life time opportunity?!?!...i would :D Thank you mick!!

On July 12, 2015, I considered myself a lucky girl. I went to my cousin's house to extract honey from beehives. Liquid gold. I believe honey works wonders in a medicinal sense. Not to mention it's pretty tasty too.

Facebook Post July 12, 2015:
What a lovely Sunday morning to be extracting honey from beehives

I had been drinking a lot of water with honey. I used to add it to my bottled water. One day I was hanging out in my aunt's yard and finished the water from the water bottle but there was honey caked to the bottom. I felt inclined to hold the water bottle up toward the Sun and look through it like a kaleidoscope. I noticed that when I looked through the water bottle with one eye it was the same color as the blonde honey or a yellowish color. When I looked through with the other eye it looked like the amber colored honey. Right at that point, the song "Amber" by 311 resonated in my mind. "Amber is the color of your energy...whooaa." My mind was doing flips. And I was doing handstands. I felt so full of energy and empowered that it was like my body couldn't contain the energy. Popping handstands and doing crunches throughout the day was a good release for me.

Facebook Post July 13, 2015:
My 1990s fanny pack > any purse ever made

Facebook Post July 13, 2015:
I wanna take it back to the hippie days....PEACE. LOVE. & ROCK n' ROLL

Peace. Love. Rock n' Roll. I thought my ideas were brilliant. One idea was to start instilling the Golden Rule back into the mindset of the human race. "Treat others the way you would like to be treated." That's a good start at peace, right? I remember the Golden Rule being displayed in my classrooms growing up. I thought, why not post it in present day classrooms? It was just an idea and I figured you have to start somewhere. Something told me that trying to positively influence children was a good place to start. Frederick Douglass said, "It's easier to build strong children than to repair broken men." Now I'm not saying to ignore issues in older cohorts. I'm just saying that raising respectful, strong, kind, caring and honest children is one avenue to take in the mission for peace. Everyone fights their own battles, there's no reason to make things worse when peace is a better way.

Facebook Post July 13, 2015:

I hope you will take a moment to read: some may think it's crazy for me to share this but my only purpose for doing so is to help others out there...no doubt others fight their own battles on a daily basis...something we often forget...well im here to let others out there know you're not alone...I hit ROCK BOTTOM back in Fall 2013...I was a NOBODY...I took nothing in - nothing went out...but with the undying care, support and love of my immediate/extended family, dogs, friends and counselors...I am soooooooo PROUD AND GRATEFUL to say that I am moving up this mountain...I feel sooo amazing these days...in fact, im sprinting. HOOYAH! So I urge others to use the power of conversation- whether it's with self, nature, family, friend, pet or fellow citizen...in company with music and dance, my personal crutch these days, to help get all the negative energy built up inside - OUT!... let out the negative, focus on being positive during every moment no matter what it may be, RESPECT - treat others the way you would like to be treated - KARMA!... choose your crutch wisely...KEEP YOUR HEAD UP, LOVE...and chances are...GREAT things will come...at least its been working for me. PEACE!

Radiate positivity. This became my new mantra. The power of positivity and capturing positive vibes from others creates a happiness within oneself. And I wanted to spread that message and those vibes.

Facebook Post July 14, 2015:

I think Disney movies are special...Walt has crazy positive vibes/energy that he feeds to the world...some people are lucky enough to catch those vibes and actually live through one of his fairytales...im pretty sure I sniped some of his vibes...never gonna let these vibes go...ill be bathing UNDER THE SEA for the rest of my life ...oh and one more thing I also feel your lucky enough to feel other stories too. If you dig deep enough into nature...ease that mind and let energy guide you...and I will leave whoever is reading this with these words...And I don't think I chose them wisely...I feel I chose them wisely...

Hakuna Matata Everyone...Think HAPPY THOUGHTS...we can all fly together...c'mon though for real...WE got the WHOLE WORLD IN OUR HANDS...ok I'm done...time to rest my eyes...If my happy little mind would let me!

Dee dee...duh deet...THAT'S ALL FOLKS!

My Facebook posts were like an insight into how manic my mind was becoming. Looking back on them now, they're like a road map tracing the path of my manic episode. The more manic I became, the more frequent, lengthy and unhinged the posts became.

Facebook Post July 14, 2015:
"Get up, stand up: stand up for your rights!

Get up, stand up: stand up for your rights!

Get up, stand up: stand up for your rights!

Get up, stand up: don't give up the fight!..."

-"Get Up Stand Up" by Bob Marley

ON A MISSION...Hoping I can recruit some people to join me on this fight for respect and peace. I have some great ideas to help Buffalo, US and

WORLD...to be a better way! And I won't back down---thanks to my man, Tom Petty and his vibes!

Peace. Love. Happiness...I wanna be there...let's go! Hopefully I can encourage others to grab their saddles...and GIDDY UP with me!

ONE DAY!

Facebook Post July 14, 2015:
I cannot believe the amount of people that have reached out to me in the past 24 hrs...But you all have me on Cloud 9. Can't get enough of this NATURAL high I'm feeling these days...but nobody, nobody is taking it from me... it's way to good...I mean c'mon..I feel like a Queen!...fer real tho...keep radiating those positive vibes people. Rain or shine...oh, and SNOW of course. peace and love.

Facebook Post July 14, 2015:
Always thought my initials were comical...for Bull Shit...but now...I see it different...in a more half glass full type mentality...perhaps...Buffalo Soldier?!

Facebook Post July 14, 2015:
Its crazy...so many musicians and artists out there...have soo much soul... they felt the vibes im feeling now a long time ago...we stopped letting Mother Nature carry us and started THINKING TOO MUCH...not just too much but too much about money and power. MONEY DOES NOT BUY HAPPINESS..in fact I DISLIKE money...and look at the mess this world is in...its time to melt this toxic snowman down...and rebuild a snowman like Buffalonians know how...taking in these vibes from this song right now! (link posted for video of "What's Going On"- Marvin Gaye)...urge others to as well...and not for anything who doesn't have a few minutes to honor and enjoy a great musician...and we all heard it before its only on T.V. every other day...

"LIFE MOVES PRETTY FAST IF YOU DON'T STOP AND LOOK AROUND ONCE IN AWHILE YOU COULD MISS IT"...Cheers to you, Marvin!

Facebook Post July 14, 2015:

This girl is like my best friend, but doesn't know it...All she's helped me through over the YEARS...hope to one day have to opportunity to tell her again, but next time, in person...Preferably on the Ellen show! Now I'm dreaming! But who said a girl can't dream...(crossing foot over)....ANNNN-NNNYYYWWAAAAYYYYY,

Grateful Alecia, for your support, inspiration..and most importantly... PINK! Sending positive vibes and a trillion Thank You's your way...(posted with link of the "Don't Let Me Get Me" by Pink)

Facebook Post July 14, 2015:

Starting to realize that best friends are not necessarily supposed to last forever... at least consecutively...embrace the camaraderie...flow naturally... make new friends... BUT KEEP THE OLD...nothin like a childhood friend-ship...and if your patient and positive...your SOULMATE...will naturally end up right by your side...and your soulmate..well lasts forever of course... but don't you dare forget about those best friends, because that they still are... and if you continue to wait patiently life will bring You and your SOUL-MATE, RIGHT BACK TO YOUR BEST FRIENDS front door...and you know who they are...because when you cross paths later in life, no matter how long its been, you pick right back up as if you were just coolin' with each other the day before on a front porch swing!

Facebook Post July 15, 2015:

PEACE MOVEMENT- I AM ON A MISSION...TO LEAVE BEHIND THE WORLD A BETTER WAY! LET US ALL WORK TOGETHER— through greed, money and power- and straight up, NEGATIVE ENERGY...

because without positive energy…Our Spirits die…and in turn the world be-comes a TOXIC place… it is time we start paying Our Ancestors a favor for watching over us all these years…LIFT UP THEIR SPIRITS—as well as your own by- throwing up high fives, peace signs, hugs, smiles, laughs, DANC-ING, SINGING…WE AS A WORLD NEED TO START RADIATING POS-ITIVE ENERGY…thru and thru—most importantly too KEEP CALM while doing so…no matter how hard the struggle- CARRY ON- Let your past be the sound of your feet upon the ground…GIDDY UP!...and through the MENTALITY of the GOLDEN RULE: TREAT OTHERS THE WAY YOU WOULD LIKE TO BE TREATED…which in NATURALITY is how it should be…WE AS A WORLD NEED TO START RESPECTING- Self, Others and most importantly, Mother Nature. If you stick with me you'll NEVER GO HUNGRY AGAIN!!! But what WILL happen…there will be blue skies, sunshine, rainbows, crazy cool designed clouds, butterflies, frogs on bongos, sunflowers, rain dances…IGLOOS and you CAN NOT FORGET THOSE SWEET HONEY BEES! It is time to melt down this toxic Snowman that has been wreaking havoc on this world for a decade if not more…KEEP ME CALM—TRUST ME IT IS SOOO IMPORTANT I STAY CALM…but please consider joining me on this journey in rebuilding the World…one of Our Greatest Gifts From OUR God…maybe drop me a like? If you are with me and want to be the change in the world, leave behind the world a better way… for those who follow…ya know PAY IT FORWARD MENTALITY…I AM STARTING TO REBUILD A POSITIVE FROSTY THE SNOWMAN, ya know, one with a Jolly Happy Ol' Soul…In fact already started, but the thing is I CAN NOT DO THIS ALL…Teamwork My Fellow Citizens…and the only response I need to this message is all in your actions…DON'T WORRY BE HAPPY…and SOMEWHERE OUT THERE…OVER THAT RAINBOW… BLUE BIRDS FLY—and I wonder why oh why can't I…but it took me 29 years to learn to use my greatest gift and I can not help but want to share this gift of mine with the WHOLE WORLD—work toward making it a GREEN WORLD AFTER ALL…and by green I DO NOT MEAN TOXIC MONEY— which kills our trees…I mean MOTHER NATURE—embrace Her, Respect

Her, Great things will come! It is all about a perfect balance- Yin and Yang... Mark my words but stand by me, my actions! Pinky Promise.

R.E.S.P.E.C.T

PEACE. LOVE. HAPPINESS. and...

ETERNAL SUNSHINE OF THE SPOTLESS MIND...Jump on My Peace Train! Think happy thoughts, learn to fly, feel the positive vibes and embrace those vibes—they are Loved ones...trust me!

GRACIAS, Mother Mary, for standing by me all these years! I wanna make you...PROUD MARY!! (posted with a link of "Proud Mary" by Tina Turner)

My excessive Facebook posts over the course of a couple of days, including quantity, length, and content, along with my lack of sleep and elated mood, had raised more concerns for my family. For as erratic as my posts had become, I was behaving even more manic and strange in person. I would begin talking a mile a minute about each new idea that would come into my mind. And it would often come out as a jumbled and confusing rant to my family. I would hop from one topic to the next, wanting to enlighten them on all the wonderful ideas and associations that were racing rapidly through my mind. I also began collecting random objects from around the house like a spider-man stuffed animal, coffee mugs, photos, and building "shrines" with them. And proudly explaining to everyone in detail what each object represented. Needless to say, my increasingly erratic and bizarre behavior became alarming to my family. They worried I might be slipping into another episode and sat down with me to express their concerns and said that they wanted to take me to Lakeshore Behavioral Health to be evaluated. To them, it was clear that something wasn't right, but to me I was feeling great and energized and better than I had felt in months. So, I was resistant to their concerns and believed I was fine. Below is a letter my family wrote to me to communicate their concerns in an effort to get me help, once again.

Dear B,

I'm glad you asked us to write things down for you to read. I think it is a better way for us to communicate without you feeling like you're being attacked or ganged up on. I can see that when we've tried to talk to you, you're hurt by it and that is the last thing we want. We love you so much and want what is best for you always.

These last few months you have seemed to be getting back to your old self again and that has made me so happy. I think you're right when you say that those months right when you got out of the hospital were kind of like you were in a fog/ not really there. B you don't know how much I missed "the old B" during that time. The energetic, hilarious, caring person that we all know. I want you to read something that I had on my computer that I wrote last July following your first episode when you were still heavily medicated and out of it. It was such a hard time for all of us and I found that writing things down helped me sometimes. I wrote this about a dream I had about you during that time:

--I had a dream about B last night and I haven't been able to stop thinking about it since. It was one of those dreams that is so vivid that even in waking life you continue to have mental images of it pop up in your head. Almost as if it were a memory instead of a dream. As if it actually happened. It was also one of those dreams where you wish it did happen. Where you lie there after just waking up, feeling happy, until the realization washes over you that it's not real.

B appeared. But not present-day B. This was B pre-break. B: in shape, doing handstands against the wall, lights in her eyes, alert, hyper, responsive, life of the party B. She looked at me intently, looked into my eyes and asked eagerly, "Where did you go? Where did you guys go from my life?" It was like she was back from a long trip. Back from being away for a while. But she was home now, all at once, altogether, and wholly the person she was before. The one who I remember. The one who I grew up with, shared a room with for 18 years of my life.

The next part of the dream is less vivid but involved Carlie being there and being really excited and explaining to B that she was coming back to us now. And within a few days the whole thing would be completely healed. Everything would be back to normal and this entire nightmare would be over and forgotten.

After that I woke up. I woke up feeling so happy and hopeful. The dream was sort of like a wish-fulfillment for me because I want it to be that simple. I want all of this to be healed and back to normal at once. But it is not simple and it is not easy. It's clear that even coming off the medication, B isn't going to come back to us like that overnight. It's not going to be just a healthy vision of her former self showing up one day and asking what the hell happened and where we've all been. I honestly don't know what is going to happen and my fear is that we'll never get her back fully. Obviously, that is horrible and pessimistic and I avoid thinking that way because it's important to remain positive, but sometimes it creeps in.

I think the reason the dream affected me so much was because we've been dealing with these changes so gradually for months. Obviously, the initial break was drastic. But the recovery since then has been subtle changes over time. So, to see the old B show up like that and be talking to me was jarring. Like seeing a ghost or something. Or like the old B was sent away, completely unaware of the pain and misery going on here, replaced with someone else, and now she was back and asking what happened. That seems callous to describe it like that. I know. That's still my sister upstairs and I don't forget that. It's just that I don't let it show, but deep down I'm mourning the loss of the sister I knew before. It's like a person died and was replaced with someone similar but not quite the same. I know it's B in there. I love her. So much. She needs us and I will not give up on her. Ever. But sometimes I just miss her.--

I wanted you to read that because I want you to understand why we're voicing our concerns to you right now. It's because we love you so much and after everything happened with ECMC two years ago, it took such a long time to get you back. That was so painful to go through and to watch you go through. We just got you back, and I don't want to lose you again, B. So, now we are doing everything in our power to not let it get to that point again.

I want you to understand that we're not saying any of this to you to try to change you in any way or to try and bring you down. I know you're feeling amazingly positive right now. Don't get me wrong – that is a good thing. I love that you're so positive and full of energy. And I think you're handling everything with Paul leaving amazingly well.

The thing is that now we're starting to see some signs that are reminiscent of the last time this all started. I know this is the part you don't want to hear. But you have to understand B that after everything happened last time, we all made sure to educate ourselves on what to look for so that we could prevent it from happening again. I realize that what you're feeling right now seems normal to you. But your behavior and thoughts two years ago also probably seemed normal to you at the time. It wasn't until you were well again that you could see things clearly. Think of what could have been avoided if we had intervened earlier last time. We could have avoided ECMC altogether. Well now we know better and that's why we're speaking up. I'm just asking you to trust us B. Is there anyone in this world that you trust more than your family? We know you better than anyone and so when we see these subtle things that others, and maybe even you, don't see, then we need to point them out.

I know you keep saying that you're not having paranoia or delusions- you're right, and that's the whole point. It hasn't gotten that bad yet and that is good because that means we still have time to get it under control. And that's all we're trying to do. I think maybe when we talk to you about these things you get worried that we're suggesting the same course of action as last time (extended stay at ECMC and two years on debilitating meds). That's not what we're suggesting at all – that is what we're trying to prevent. We're not suggesting some drastic action. All we want is for all of us to go and see someone together and help us figure this out. They say the most important thing in situations like these is to be proactive instead of reactive. Not wait for something to happen. And that's all we're trying to do.

So please, for your sake and for the sake of our family please just be open to what we're trying to say. Don't take it as us trying to bring you down or change you. We're trying to keep you as positive and high energy as you've always been, because we don't want to see you down and hurting again. Please don't get upset and please try to understand that sometimes in these situations, the people who love us can see things that we ourselves can't always see.

The letter was compelling and heartfelt, but unfortunately after reading it, I still didn't believe I needed help. I was so manic and far gone at that point that I just couldn't see things clearly. Looking back at it now and reading the letter, it makes me realize the desperation my family was feeling and makes me feel bad that at the time I wasn't capable of receiving it and comprehending it the way I should've. I couldn't see what they were seeing. At that point I was already in such a manic state of mind that I wasn't able to recognize the signs that they were seeing and wasn't able to respond appropriately to their concerns.

Even though the letter didn't have the intended effect, my family continued to talk to me and try to reason with me and persuade me to go to Lakeshore. Finally, I gave in and I said that I would go, but only if I got to meet with my old chemical dependency counselor. She was a counselor I had come to trust and who had helped me a lot in our sessions in the past. She was easy to talk to and gave good advice. Unfortunately, when my family called Lakeshore we were informed that she was out of the country at the time, in Budapest. The song "Budapest" by George Ezra came to my mind and I pulled up the YouTube video to listen to that song and lit up a cigarette. My mind started wandering with thought. As I was smoking it dawned on me. I started to think that the real reason my family wanted me to go to Lakeshore was to help my mother and I quit smoking. Especially my mother. So finally, I gave in and agreed to go to Lakeshore. As I paced around the house waiting to leave, I started to come across objects throughout the house that had deep meaning to me. I gathered together the meaningful items which I wanted to use as props in the meeting with the counselors. These items consisted of, but were not limited to: a rosary, toy figurines - one which included Chuckie from the children's cartoon "Rugrats," candy, playing cards, tweezers, a wine cork, honey, a pink mini porcupine ball that represented Pink, the singer, and a lime green porcupine ball that represented Ellen Degeneres, a globe, and a Virgin Mary Statue. Each item represented something to me. And I felt I needed to tell the story behind the objects to the counselors at Lakeshore. I put on what I thought was my best outfit for spreading positivity: a black t-shirt with the words Vision, Passion and Power written in rainbow letters, which I had bought in the past from the Rock and Roll Hall of Fame honoring women in music; I also wore tall black socks with colorful peace signs and hot pink trim, topped off with my salmon colored "Fifel Goes West" hat with a diamond butterfly broach clipped to it. And of course, my sunglasses - because I felt I could not look anyone directly in the eyes except my family. (This was probably a sign that paranoid thoughts were starting to develop in my mind). Needless to say, my eccentric outfit - which was very symbolic and meaningful to me, drew some raised eyebrows and chuckles from my family.

My mind was moving at a rapid pace, and jumping from thought to thought, so my thinking wasn't entirely linear at the time. Lakeshore is located near my cousin's house. So, as we were getting ready to leave, my mind shifted. I went from thinking we were going to Lakeshore to get help for my mom and I, to the idea that we were actually going to my cousin's house for a big party. I proceeded to fill the car that we would be taking with a variety of different items for the party. These items included a kids-sized electric organ, my guitar, two giant rainbow pinata 8's to represent #88 Patrick Kane, along with the rest of the items I had collected. Relating back to my first episode, sports players held a lot of weight in creating positivity. I enlisted the help of my sisters and my cousin to carry these items outside and load them into the car. I'm sure they were very confused about my reasoning especially given the randomness of the items, but they humored me anyway.

Once everything was jam packed into the car, everyone squeezed around the assortment of items. I was excited about the idea of going to the party, but as we were driving my family reminded me that we were going to Lakeshore. I suddenly remembered that we were going there to help my mother and I quit smoking. And since Lakeshore was on the way to my cousin's house, I agreed to make the stop there, figuring we would just be going to the party afterwards.

When we arrived at Lakeshore, we were directed to the more private waiting room that did not have any other patients in there. I paced around the waiting room anxiety-ridden. I stepped outside to have a cigarette and I noticed a flyer hanging on the window that said "OASAS." The first thing that crossed my mind was the song "Wonderwall" by Oasis. For some reason I associated "Wonderwall" with Kane #88 of the Chicago Blackhawks. More specifically, the lyrics "because maybe, you're gonna be the one that saves me," and the idea that his abilities as a professional sports player could produce positivity by scoring the final goal in a game and getting a victory. To me, this was a matter of being able to create positivity on a big scale - a life-changing scale. For example, as mentioned during my first episode, I felt that by scoring goals and winning games, he had the ability to actually save people's lives from situations such as terrorist attacks and natural disasters. He had the ability to save people from dying.

I returned to the waiting room. I had brought a small stick in with me from outside. It had caught my eye because I thought it resembled the center of a peace sign. So, I picked it up from the ground before returning to the waiting room. I believed I could use the stick to "zap" people in order to give them positive vibes. I was soon called back to a conference room to meet with a counselor named Judy. I proceeded with a discussion, mainly of myself telling a story using all the props I had brought to the room. The counselors were doing their best to have me focus and to have a serious discussion. But my family tells me that instead, I was pacing back and forth at the front of the room and giving a very animated presentation to everyone about the meaning of the props. There was another counselor, Meredith, that kept entering and leaving the room. I was getting bad vibes from her. I even went as far as to tell her that her inner child was dead. At one point when she was exiting the room, I firmly pointed my stick at her in an attempt to zap her with positive vibes. Needless to say, after a brief meeting, it didn't take long for the counselors to decide that I needed to be checked into in-patient care at BryLin, a hospital for Behavioral Health. Now I was still under the impression that this was all a part of trying to get my mother and me into a program that would assist us with smoking cessation. So, I agreed to go. I was happy to do it for my mother.

We arrived at BryLin and entered the intake office. It was a really small room, with a small desk and a couple of chairs. While waiting to be signed in, I grew overly excited and anxious. Due to these overwhelming feelings, I lost control of my bladder and I peed my pants. The nurse got me a pair of "Depends" disposable underwear and a smock to change into. The nurse began with some questions and started with, "Who are you?" With a chuckle I replied, "Who am I?" In rapid-fire succession I began to give the nurse all the titles I had proudly given myself. "My name is B. Amber Stark, I am an optimistic realist, nature embracer, positive peacemaker, energizer bunny, queen B, Buffalo Soldier, and now..." At that point, I paused and dramatically lifted up my smock and revealed the "Depends" underwear I was wearing and shouted, "TOOOMMMY PICKLES" as I shook my hips to emphasize my resemblance to the diapered "Rugrats" character. The room, which was filled with my family - mom, dad, sisters, my cousin, a family friend and the nurse, erupted into laughter. I was pretty enthusiastic with my introduction and my family tells me that it was a much-needed moment of levity during an otherwise tense time.

Following the intake questions, it was determined that I needed to stay in the hospital. I was suffering from a manic state and needed to be monitored and prescribed medication. Partly because I was in such an elated state that I could have been a risk to others and/or myself. My feeling of being invincible was a concern. In the mind of someone with mania, there are no limits to what one can do, considering grandiosity and invincibility are hallmarks of mania. So, it was best for me to be contained and prescribed the proper medication to bring me back to reality. I was escorted to my room.

There wasn't really a whole lot to do. So, pacing became a favorite activity just like at ECMC. Not to mention I was loaded with energy from the mania. The hall I was staying in was in a "T" shape. I would constantly pace the floor in the "T" formation. One thing I noticed immediately about BryLin were the positive and uplifting paintings on the walls throughout the floor. The pictures made this "home away from home" more comforting. There were two main larger common areas to hang out in, and one smaller one. The smaller one was only allowed to have so many people in it at a time. This room was referred to as the "calming room." It had books and a big recliner chair inside. And music! The best part was the music. So, I would find myself in this room a lot throughout my stay.

I remember that before I arrived at the hospital my thoughts were not paranoid. I was just extremely happy and felt extremely energetic and invincible. My mind was moving a mile a minute and thoughts were just racing by. I was making associations left and right. Things were coming to mind that I hadn't thought of in a long time. Songs, movies, people. I loved to tell others what was on my mind. I believed that the spirits of those who had passed guided people in present day. And the more positive energy that was produced in the world, the more our late loved ones' souls could help us. They were never really gone.

My memories from BryLin are meshed together and are not really linear or in sequential order. I am not sure when certain events, behaviors and thoughts occurred. I just remember them happening. However, I am able to categorize my experiences according to the first room I stayed in and the second room I stayed in at the hospital. I will do my best to present them in a coherent sequence.

It's important to note that although my thoughts were not really paranoid at the beginning, throughout my stay my thoughts did grow paranoid. The type of paranoia I experienced in my first episode consisted of terrified paranoia in which I felt helpless and utterly terrified about everything. We were doomed, and everything was a life and death situation. Life was being lost in my mind. The type of paranoia I experienced at BryLin during this second episode consisted of fear, but in a different capacity. I believe my mania and feeling of being invincible led me to believe that I had the ability to overcome the fear. So, instead of cowering down in a corner and tiptoeing around a "life and death situation," I walked right into each paranoid situation head-on with the idea that I had the means to get through it. Now mind you these were all phantom delusions. Reality with a twist. The paranoias and beliefs I had simply did not exist. But to me they were real.

I remember being placed in a room midway down the hallway that had an adjoining bathroom with the room next to it. I was in a room by myself so there was a single bed. My family needed to bring me clothes since I needed to stay until further notice. I finished getting situated and waited for my parents to come back up to the hospital with the rest of my stuff. I was a little more comfortable being at BryLin than I was at ECMC. Mainly because I was perceiving everything in a different way due to my state of mind. ECMC was scary to me right from the beginning because I had already been in that paranoid mindset before even going to the hospital. At BryLin I was on cloud nine and was loving life at the beginning so everything seemed more positive right from the get-go.

While I waited for my family, the nurses had me fill out the visitor's permission form, which was a list of names I had to provide to the hospital of who I wanted to be allowed to visit me. In the meantime, my friend Rhee came to visit me. She brought me a coconut water, which was my "go-to" drink at the time, and a Rafiki beanie baby, which is a character from the Lion King. We were sitting at the table in one of the visitors' rooms. A nurse approached and asked how I was doing. I picked up my coconut water and replied referencing the Lion King character Zazu's version of the lyrics from the song "I've Got A Lovely Bunch Of Coconuts." I felt like I was channeling Walt Disney's vibes. My friend and I shared a chuckle.

My family arrived with clothes and slippers for me. One of the nurses informed my family that they might want to update my visitors list because their names hadn't made it onto the list that I filled out and turned in. Puzzled as to who I had put on the list, they asked to see it. The nurse showed them the list I made, which consisted of the following three people: Pink, Ellen Degeneres and my friend, Rhee. I was under the impression that family was automatically allowed and that the visitor list was needed for non-family members only.

I took a quick shower while my family waited for me to get out. I was nervous to do it without them there. I freshened up and put some clean clothes on. They brought me something to eat and we visited briefly.

I spent the next couple of hours scoping out the floor, passing by new floormates with a smile. I felt like I knew why I was there. The feeling was all too familiar yet new at the same time. I was there to radiate positive vibes. Flip negative into positive. Again.

It was 9:00 PM and time for meds. Bedtime was approaching. I had a racing mind. It made for a rough night's sleep. But I made it. I grabbed my

Rafiki beanie baby, the blanket my family brought for me and I dozed off.

Now I don't recall being totally unstable until after I started the medication at the hospital. Beforehand, I was just uber excited about life and people and radiating positivity and love; just straight up ecstatic. Yes, my thoughts were racing, but in an organized fashion. It wasn't until the next day or two that I started to think irrational thoughts.

One activity I engaged in a lot was coloring. One night I could not sleep so I was coloring in the dining area with one of the other patients. I was taken aback because she chose to color a picture of a cat and a dog. Without me even saying anything to her, she decided to color the dog the same color as my childhood dog and the cat the same color as my childhood cat. I took this as a sign. It was as if she was channeling my former pets' souls or spirits. I saved the picture she colored to add to my collection of pictures. Not only did I enjoy coloring pictures, but other patients on the floor would color pictures with me and I would save them. I often found myself in the calming room listening to music while I colored. One night specifically, I colored with Carol Ann. I called her Carol Ann because she reminded me of Carol Ann from the movie *Poltergeist*. I thought I had to increase positive interaction with her. She had a hearing aid and my paranoid thoughts had me thinking it was really a device used for outside communication telling her what to say to me and listening to our conversations.

I used the collection of colored images from coloring books, which had meaning to me, to create a shrine in my first room. I laid the pictures across the room in a sequenced order, ranging from my closet and reaching all the way across the floor to my bed which was on the opposite side of the room. The first picture in the shrine was a picture of an excited dog eating out of a bowl. On the front of the bowl I wrote, "On A Mission." The pictures were placed in a specific order that told a story and I referred to the train of images as my "Peace Train." Pertaining to my mission for peace. And making the world a better way. As I looked at the shrine, I realized the pictures divided my room into positive and negative spaces.

Unfortunately, the positive space was the smaller section between the bed, wall, and shrine. The negative space was the rest of the room outside the shrine wall. I used to do handstands inside the positive space in an effort to expand the positive energy in the room. I would do a handstand in the positive space and slowly lower my legs down into the negative space as if I was transmitting the positive vibes from the positive space to the negative space. I remember one day I found one of the nurses checking on my room to see if I was in there. I came in behind her and she said I had to clean up the shrine. I begged her to let me leave it because it exuded positivity.

Aside from the coloring book pictures, there was also a towel that my family brought in for me and I thought there was a purpose for them bringing it in. The towel had three frogs with happy expressions on their faces, staggered across the towel on lily pads. I thought the towel represented my three sisters. So, I hung the towel on the outside of my closet at the one end of the shrine in my room. This towel possessed a lot of positivity. And it was my duty to protect it, or in my mind, them - my sisters. Sometimes I would lie in the bed with the towel over me. It comforted me and made me feel as if my sisters were there with me in spirit.

I remember panicking on the inside at one point while I was assigned to my first room. I was in fear that my sister, Carlie, was in danger. I believed she had been hurt at work and was being cared for at the same hospital on another floor. At this point my thoughts and behaviors had become extremely irrational. I thought she was on a breathing machine in the hospital. So, I scurried to my room with a straw. A side note, I would walk around the floor with my Rafiki beanie baby tied to the string of my pants. At that point I thought I could use the Rafiki beanie baby to save my sister. At first, I was afraid that the string was tied too tight around him which translated to my sister's circulation being cut off. I quickly untied him. Then I proceeded to take the straw, line it up with Rafiki's mouth and blow into the straw. I continued to do this as I paced around my room. I was trying to breathe life back into my sister.

My other sister, Ava, had brought me my locket that had a picture inside of my late great aunt and me. It was a gift she had given to me after my great aunt had passed away. I remember wearing it one night and it sounded like it was ticking. I kept bringing it to my ear and it was for sure ticking like a time bomb. At least I thought so. Hallucination. I was overcome with fear and ripped the necklace off my neck and threw it in the garbage. Unfortunately, I never got the locket back which is a regret I still have to this day.

I also noticed wads of black hair on the floor in my room. I got down on my knees and stared at the wads of hair. They literally looked like they were moving. Hallucination. I was overcome with fear as I thought the hair was some sort of computerized germ being controlled by enemies. I thought the hair would crawl through the orifices of my body while I was sleeping and cause me ailments such as paranoia and hallucinations. So, I picked the wads of hair up with a tissue and flushed them down the toilet.

My bathroom was connected to another patient's room. One day I remember feeling like I was being followed, so I was afraid to exit the bathroom through my side of the bathroom. So instead, I went through the connecting patient's room. Patients are not allowed to go into other patients' rooms without permission. At that point, the nurses decided to switch me to a room that had a bathroom that did not connect to another patient's room. This room was next to the showers at the end of the hallway, at the opposite end of the hallway from the nurses' station. My mind was racing with thoughts. Different scenarios and situations were criss-crossing around in my head.

By the time I was moved to my second room, my previous thought processes from my first episode had revisited me. The idea of needing to radiate positive energy was getting stronger. My ability to sleep was decreasing. I was often strolling down to the nurse's station at late hours of the night. And again, at early hours in the morning.

There was a camera at the end of the hallway near the nurse's station. It tracked activity all the way down the hallway to my new room. I thought I was being watched through the camera to the point that I thought a movie was being made using the footage of me. I remember I would walk down the hall late at night since I couldn't sleep. I would walk along the walls to avoid being in the center of the camera. Another reason I did this was due to the fact that I thought I was being tracked and I thought I was going to be struck by a laser. I thought a laser would be sent from the camera lens. After several times walking down the hallway I had it in my mind that it was easier for the laser to target me if I walked in a straight line. Therefore, whenever I would walk down the hall I would zig-zag from one side to the other. I figured it was harder to hit a moving target.

One particular night I found myself in the dining area very late. Everyone else on the floor was asleep. Everyone but me, of course. I sat with one of the nurses who made me think of Harriet Ross Tubman. I really thought it might have been her. A younger version of her. Like she had aged backwards. I called her Harriet. But we sat at the table and I told her the story of everything that happened to me right up until entering BryLin. I gave her insight on the history of my first episode and what was happening in my life leading up to my first episode. As we sat and talked, a random thought popped into my head about the rapper DMX, or "Uncle," as I referred to him in my first episode. At the time, DMX actually happened to be at the Erie County Holding Center which was nearby. It had been in the news that he had been there. I thought he was going to show up that night at the hospital. And I was going to have to talk to him. I didn't know why he was at the holding center but I figured it was for something negative and it needed to be made positive.

There was a peculiar man that would come to the floor occasionally. I don't know if he was a worker at the hospital, or if he was another patient's visitor, but he used to sit in a chair somewhere along the hallway and he would always be reading. One idea I had in my mind was that we were being attacked by China. And the camera on the wall by the nurses' station was actually a live feed to the world. People around the world supported me in my efforts to radiate positivity and fight off the negative energy. It was a reminder that radiating positivity on the floor translated to creating positive situations in the outside world. I believed that because I have Irish roots, this meant that Ireland was "on my side." Therefore, I thought this man, who I believed was Irish, was there to indirectly help me get through my stay and get out of the hospital. I saw that he was reading all the time so I felt that he was trying to tell me to read. Reading would inform me of the outside world and help me to act in a manner that would make the world a better way. I remember taking a stack of books from the calming room and putting them in my room. I spent about an hour going back and forth, picking out books with titles that stood out to me, and placing them on the shelf in my closet. After I was done setting them up, I was nervous I was going to get in trouble for putting the books in my room. So, I proceeded to return them back to the calming room, and returned to my room with just one. I was reading the book and a "formula" popped into my head. I was supposed to read the first three pages, the middle three pages and the last three pages. I believed I would get the most important information from these pages. I thought that time was of the essence and in my mind, I needed to get the best information that I could in a short amount of time. I remember reading part of a story that was about two men that approached a door to someone's house. These were bad guys and were out to hurt this particular person. I immediately thought of my friend, Rhee, and I thought that story was telling me to help her. So, I ran to the phone. I called her and told her not to answer her door if someone comes to her house. I told her to just trust me not to answer the door. She sounded confused but said, "okay."

I had a nightly routine of making my way to the nurses' station. One night when I got down to the nurses' station, I realized one of the other patients was sitting in the recreation room at the ping-pong table. So, I decided to join her. I told her I was going to get a coffee cocktail and asked if she wanted anything. She agreed to a coffee. So, I went and made myself a cup of half coffee and half hot water, with a packet of hot cocoa mix. And I got her a coffee with cream and sugar. We sat there at the table and talked for hours about our situations. She was a little older and had experienced mental health ailments in the past. So, she gave me some insight on how to deal with it as well as how to deal with some issues I was having in my personal life. Eventually we grew sleepy and went to bed.

I should note that the little kitchen area had a coffee/tea station. The machine had a red and green light on it. I thought these lights were lasers and was afraid that the bad guys were going to try and shoot me with the lasers. So, whenever I would go in there, it was very calculated. I would only stay in there for less than a minute at a time and I would walk along the kitchen counter "out of the line of fire" of the laser.

Another thing I started doing was heating tea bags and then rubbing the tea bag on my face. I felt the herbal properties of the tea were good for my skin. I remember one day the nurse (who I thought was Ellen Degeneres' brother) asked me what was on my face. My face would have a tea-stained color on it. I told him that it had benefits from the herbal properties in the tea and that I thought it was good for my skin.

I remember requesting that my family bring me my peacock sneakers to wear, which were sneakers that had peacock feather designs all over them. I wanted them to bring me the sneakers so that I'd have better traction if I needed to run away from a bad guy. I was afraid that the slippers I had been wearing would be hard to run in and I wouldn't be able to get away. But, after pacing constantly for days in the sneakers, my feet began to hurt. I attributed the pain and the fact that my feet felt heavy to the peacock sneakers. With the notion that the U.S. was under attack from China, I thought that the sneakers were rigged with a bomb. And that they had a tracking device in them which China was using to track me. I thought that the energy from them tapping into the tracking device happened to be causing the sneakers to feel heavy, thus hurting my feet. I thought the pressure I was feeling was a bomb about to explode. I also thought if I took the sneakers off, it would prevent China from tracking me and prevent the bomb from being detonated. So, I threw the sneakers in a paper bag and closed the bag. I called my parents and asked them to bring me my superhero rainboots instead when they came to visit. I thought my superhero boots were comprised of positive energy. I had worn them at the

Bonnaroo Music and Arts Festival in Tennessee one year and I felt they had "bonnaroovian" qualities. From my experience, Bonnaroo is a very positive and happy place so I thought the boots contained that same energy. When my parents arrived, I took the boots and gave them the bag with the peacock sneakers and told them to throw them away.

I remember running into an issue with running out of clean clothes at the hospital. I would cycle through the clothes my parents brought up for me so quickly because I used to wear layers. So, I would end up wearing all of the clean clothes they brought to me over a matter of a couple days. Every patient had a brown bag by the door to their room. Each patient would fill the brown bag with dirty laundry and someone would come around and collect it to be cleaned. I remember filling my bag and having it picked up but I didn't have clean clothes to change into the one day. I called my friend Rhee and told her that I ran out of clothes and was waiting for the clean laundry to come back. I just wanted to shower but couldn't until I got the clean clothes back. Rhee surprised me and brought me some clothes and lotion. I went through the bag she brought me and realized she had put a giraffe t-shirt that said "What's Up?" on it in the bag. My face lit up because my signature karaoke song and one of my favorite songs of all time is "What's Up?" by 4 Non Blondes. Also, when I used to see my old counselor, she used to have giraffe pictures and miniature statues in her office. She told me that the giraffes were her favorite animal at the zoo and she used to go and see them all the time. I felt it was a sign, a way of my friend Rhee letting me know that she had talked to my old counselor and that my old counselor was there in spirit. I also thought it meant that my old counselor was going to help me at the hospital. This just goes to show how every little thing I crossed paths with had deep meaning. Nothing was superficial.

I informed Rhee that I had put the Rafiki beanie baby she'd given me in the brown bag with my dirty laundry to send it to get cleaned, but I never got it back. The next time she came to see me she brought me a little tiny giraffe stuffed animal. Like the shirt, I thought this stuffed animal was a sign that Rhee had again been in communication with my old counselor. I carried this giraffe with me at all times, all throughout the hospital floor. I thought it was powerful. I used to carry it in the center of my sports bra. From the outside of the shirt, the giraffe made three rings. It reminded me exactly of the Bonnaroo logo of three rings in the shape of a triangle. With one ring at the top center and two rings below it on either side. The nose of the giraffe made the top ring, the right arm and leg made one bottom ring and the left arm and leg made the other bottom ring. Because of this, I thought carrying the giraffe like this contributed to creating positive vibes as well as having protective properties.

I used to create things to use to my advantage, or at least what I thought was my advantage. I made a make-shift satchel out of a long-sleeved shirt. I kept items that I believed to be valuable in there, and that I did not want anyone to have access to. I would keep this bag on my person at all times, even when I would sleep. I made a make-shift doo-rag to wear on my head out of a pair of my boxer-brief underwear. I got the idea from one of the hospital workers who used to come and collect the laundry. He always had one on and I thought that I needed to do the same thing. So, I found a way. One of my pairs of underwear had flowers on it. I picked them up one day and immediately thought of the song "Flowers in Your Hair" by The Lumineers. I proceeded to put the flower underwear, which were bikini style, on my head like I did with the boxer-briefs. However, where the boxer-brief underwear looked like a doo-rag, the flower bikini underwear made me look ridiculous. I remember walking around the floor that day with the flower underwear on my head, and a doctor who resembled an older version of young Kit from the movie *A League of Their Own* saw me and asked me, "What do you have on your head?" I proudly responded, "UNDERWEAR!" She gave me a grin as if she was confused yet amused at the same time and asked me why. Seeing this doctor reinforced my suspicion that I was actually in a movie and being filmed because I was certain that this doctor was the actress from *A League of Their Own*.

I remember walking through the halls with my doo-rag on and one of the other patients, who I called David, came walking out of the kitchen wearing his tie-dye t-shirt wrapped around his head like a doo-rag. It seemed I had started a trend. I called him David because I was in the calming room one day and was reading a National Geographic magazine that had a silhouette of a man on a horse and the cover said "King David." After seeing that magazine, I noticed David as a new patient on the floor. For some reason I made the connection that he was the man on the horse from the cover. I even went as far as to show him the magazine which made him laugh. I also remember David having a really good singing voice. One morning before breakfast he sang gospel hymns to the nurses. I chimed in whenever I knew the song he was singing. Namely "Hallelujah" by Leonard Cohen. David also used to read scripture. I remember stumbling upon him reading from the Bible on a few separate occasions. David exuded positive vibes to me and his presence on the floor was a comfort to me.

Right before I entered the hospital, I was bit by a dog on my ankle while trying to break up a dog fight. I was left with holes from the teeth around my ankle. Being paranoid, I was afraid to tell anyone at the hospital about the wound. I was in fear that they were going to taint the wounds with harmful chemicals that would enter my bloodstream. So, I never mentioned the wound and would just keep it covered with tall socks.

There was a doctor I had to check in with on a weekly basis. I believed this doctor was the leader of the comic book convention, Comic Con, because his name made me think of a comic book character. So, when I went to check in with him, I made sure to wear my superhero boots. I also made sure to dress in a very colorful manner as if I were attending Comic Con. I wanted to resemble a character. I thought it would help get me discharged faster.

Similar to my first episode, I felt I was the peace against all turmoil. One morning I was in the lounge area and the Weather Channel was on T.V. Since it was really early in the morning, about 5:45 AM, the volume was low on the T.V. So, I could barely hear what was being said. But the picture displayed a big white swirl which looked like a hurricane to me. I saw this image and immediately thought I had to withstand a storm. The first thing that crossed my mind was the song "The Eye" by Brandi Carlile. The lyrics read, "you can dance in a hurricane, but only if you're standing in the eye." With these lyrics resonating in my mind, I thought there was going to be a horrible storm of negativity that I was going to be called to offset with positivity. I would have to remain calm while standing in the eye of the hurricane which would enable me to pierce through the storm and save the people of Buffalo. I remember the sky being very gloomy that day as I calmly anticipated the climax of the storm.

Outside the window of my room, I could see a huge construction vehicle parked in the lot across the street. It was parallel to where the hospital shower was located. I remember thinking that the evil forces were going to try and break through the wall of the hospital using this machine with a wrecking ball while I was in the shower, in an effort to try and kill me. Therefore, I would rush and speed-shower, as I was afraid to be in there for a long period of time.

Another issue I had with the shower was the temperature dial of the shower. You would turn the dial clockwise to turn the water on. The farther around the dial was turned, the hotter the water would be. There was a "T" imprinted on the dial, which I thought represented "Time." I thought that as I turned the dial past the "T," I would travel through time. It got to a point where I thought I would never see my family again because I thought I would travel too far in time, into the past or future. Therefore, I would quickly turn the cold water on and off enough to just wet my body. I would lather up with soap and then quickly turn it on to rinse and shut if off without passing the "T."

Every time I would take a shower, I would go to the nurses' station to get new soap. I was paranoid about using the soap that I had opened and left on my bathroom sink. I thought the soap was being laced with chemicals that would burn my skin. I wouldn't throw the bottles of soap away though. Instead, I had all the bottles lined up around the sink in my bathroom, arranged in a symmetrical fashion. It was all about balance. Balance meant positivity.

I remember looking out my window at the sun one morning. It was big and intense. I was terrified. I had this notion that China had launched a fireball towards the U.S. I, all of a sudden, went from loving the sun to thinking it was a tool of destruction headed towards the United States. Heading right towards us in slow motion. I yanked the curtains in my room shut while I stood in fear.

My parents came to visit with food as they often did. We were in the rec room where there was a pop machine. I remember my dad wanting to get a pop and I abruptly pulled his hand away from the machine and told him no. He was confused. I told him it was going to blow up if he tried to purchase a pop. He reassured me it wouldn't and proceeded to select the kind he wanted. I literally got sick on the inside as I was flooded with feelings of anxiety. But sure enough, the machine dispensed the pop without exploding.

Similar to the first episode, I was also paranoid about the food at the hospital. I was afraid to eat it. I would only eat the pre-packaged food that was offered or I would wait for my family to bring me something to eat. One particular day, I did not eat much at the hospital. Therefore, I was looking forward to my family bringing me something. They arrived and we went to the rec room and sat down. I started to open the chicken hoagie they brought me. I got up to go to the kitchen to get a plate and some napkins. When I got back my mom and dad had taken a bite of my hoagie. I was visibly upset and I told them that the devil made them do it. The devil and his negative energy because he knew I was hungry.

There were a couple of older female patients on the floor. There was one that used to carry around a stuffed buffalo. She said it brought her good luck. She would always talk to the girls on the floor in hopes of finding her son a wife. The other one was a really sweet lady who used to give me good advice and guidance. She shared a lot of words of wisdom with me randomly throughout my stay. I specifically remember her telling me that my family really loves me and that she could tell I mean a lot to them. She made the comment that I had a beautiful family. This comforted me, as did all the other wise and insightful conversations we would have. She was like a grandmother figure to me at the hospital.

Random activities and group sessions would be scheduled throughout the day. One particular activity was Zumba. I remember watching the Zumba video and mimicking the instructor on the tape. However, I added a twist to my movements. I really got into the dancing aspect of the workout. I remember on the video there were arrows that would interchange between red and green. It was almost like although we were doing the workout together, the instructors in the video were against me. So, when I saw the arrows turn red, I thought the instructors were trying to spread negative energy. Therefore, I would get really into the dance moves and thought when the arrows turned green it meant that my dance moves were working and that the negativity was being diminished and positivity was being spread.

Another thing I started to do to contribute to positive vibes was to write a positive message on the white board by the nurses' station where the date was written. I thought this was a good way to strike a good vibe with the other patients as well as the workers on the floor. One of the various sayings I would write was, "Ciao Bella!" along with a peace sign and smiley face.

An art therapy activity we engaged in one day was painting little plastic boards. They were transparent with a variety of different images. We each got to pick an image to paint. I picked an image of a giraffe by a sunset. I painted it and saved it to give to Rhee. The finished project looked like a stained-glass window with sunlight passing through the array of colors in the image. It was pretty neat.

As time went on in the hospital, I grew fearful of mirrors. So, I would often avoid looking into them, as I thought an enemy was on the other side. Not literally, but more like a camera recording a live feed through the mirror. I remember one day I had the movie *A League of Their Own* in my mind because of the one doctor who I thought was Kit from the movie. There was a mirror across from the nurses' station which I would have to walk by to get to the lounge rooms on the floor. I was approaching the mirror and thought "baseball." So, I suddenly ran really quickly and slid across the floor just beneath the mirror to avoid "being recorded and seen by the enemy."

There was a checkerboard table in the lounge where we would eat our meals. I felt that the red and black squares on the table represented negative energy. One day, right as breakfast was about to be served, I took napkins and unfolded them. I used them to cover the checkerboard table. I proceeded to take the cups provided for drinks and arranged them in a strategic manner to prevent the negative energy from growing in the room. With symmetry being a big thing for me, I arranged everything on the table in a symmetrical form. I would panic as the other patients would remove items from the table to use for the breakfast that was being served. And I would continue to rearrange the items such as the sugar bowl, the juice containers, the cups and napkins. To me, the symmetrical arrangement was comprised of positive vibes and was necessary to offset the negativity from the checkerboard table.

I found myself up late one night as usual hanging out in the café lounge. In a similar fashion to how I symmetrically arranged the items on the breakfast table, I had the urge to rearrange the tables and chairs in the form of a train. So, there I went arranging the tables and chairs into a pattern I found to be the best fit to my puzzle. I kind of envisioned being on "the train" the next morning before breakfast with the other patients on the floor. I had the two front seats of the train placed in front of the T.V. And the other chairs followed behind in a row. I, of course, would take the "driver's seat" the next morning.

In an effort to continue creating positive energy, one morning I collected newspaper articles that spoke positive vibes to me. I took the articles and displayed them across the spare table in the café lounge so everyone that entered the room would be overcome with positivity.

Several times throughout my stay, I would put jig-saw puzzles together with a few of the other patients. We would work really hard to get the puzzle done quickly. We completed a total of seven puzzles - six smaller ones and one bigger one. I cannot remember the number of pieces in each. It was a lot of fun and it was like we would rush to finish as if we were being timed. And in my mind, we were rushing to finish in order to create positivity. We would assemble the puzzles on the ping pong table in the rec room. At one point during my hospital stay I started to think that this room was filled with negative energy like the larger common area when I was at ECMC. Working together with the other patients to complete the puzzle helped to offset this negative energy. And once we were finished, we left the completed puzzles on display on one of the smaller tables in the rec room. I remember seeing both doors to the rec room shut one night. I had it in my mind that the fact that they were shut allowed for the negative energy to grow within the room. I was terrified but also felt invincible and knew I had to do something more to create positive vibes in the room. So, I mustered up the courage to go inside the rec room. In order to create positivity, I started to rearrange the puzzles symmetrically, arranging the smaller ones around the outside like a border, with the bigger puzzle in the middle.

I remember coloring a picture of three birds. After coloring the picture, I thought of the song "Put Your Records On" by Corinne Bailey Rae. In the song, the lyrics read "three little birds sat on my window and they told me I don't need to worry." The picture made me feel better and I wanted to make others feel better too. So, I decided to put the picture of the birds on display and propped the picture up on the heater against the window in the rec room. I thought this would be a way to let others know they didn't need to worry. Also, the combination of the symmetrically arranged puzzles and the picture of the birds worked together to defuse the negativity in the room.

During yet another late night, I ventured down to the nurses' station and there was another patient, a new patient, hanging out at the counter. He was in his boxer shorts and a white t-shirt. He was a bigger man and when he saw me, he referred to me as "Jesus of Nazareth." That immediately had me thinking that he was negative energy and he was the Devil and I had to work to offset his negativity. So, I engaged in small talk with him and he mentioned he was hungry. So, I directed him to the kitchen. Here I thought the best way to create positivity was to offer him food. I offered to make him a peanut butter and jelly sandwich, and he accepted. So, I happily made him a sandwich in order to keep him happy and positive. I remember as I was making the sandwich he was singing.

I noticed in the refrigerator in the kitchen there was always a lunch bag with a lock on it with one of the nurse's names on it. It was Nurse Marley's lunch bag. One day I had food left over from lunch and put it in a paper bag. I was afraid another patient or one of the nurses was going to poison my food if they knew it was mine, so I wrote Dr. Oz on the bag thinking this would prevent anyone from touching it.

Beatrice was a patient I developed a good friendship with on the floor. She was like a mother figure to me for the duration of my stay. When I was anxious, she would help talk me through it or give me a task to help redirect my mind. One day in particular I was having a rough time. She told me one thing she liked to do to help with her anxiety was to take magazines and cut out the things from the magazine that she found interest in, and then possibly work toward obtaining the items. So, I did just that. I took a magazine and cut out pictures of a collection of items and interests. Some included a bag I liked, a cellphone that was just released, a picture of a person with a hair style I liked and a watch, among other things. Engaging in this activity helped me release negative energy and calm my mind down.

One activity to help pass the time was watching movies in the café lounge. I remember one day I was hanging out in my room and ventured to the lounge to find other patients viewing a movie. I remember them telling me the movie they were watching was *Cabin Fever*. The words "cabin fever" seeped into my mind and all I could think of was getting "cabin fever" from being trapped in my room or on the same floor in the hospital for days. I'm not sure what the title *Cabin Fever* pertains to in regard to the movie but to me it meant getting deathly ill from being secluded from society in the same small space for so long.

There was a recliner chair in the calming room. I remember sitting in it one day and it felt like the arms of the chair were inflating. I thought that it was rigged with a bomb. I was afraid to get out of the chair because I thought the bomb was going to explode if I got up. So, I continued to sit there and sing the lyrics "Don't worry, about a thing, every little thing is gonna be alright" by Bob Marley until I believed I felt the arms deflate due to the positive vibes I created.

I remember seeing the cleaning lady one day with a bucket and a mop. The bucket was a yellow one on wheels. I remember seeing the wheels on the bucket and thinking of Tina Turner's version of the song "Proud Mary" (originally recorded by Creedence Clearwater Revival) and the lyrics "big wheel keep on turnin' Proud Mary keep on burnin." I realized she was "Proud Mary," like the song title, and from that point on I called her Mary.

There were phones that were made accessible to patients in the hallway of the hospital. I was afraid for the phones at the hospital to be hung up after a call. I thought that a plane was going to explode every time the phone was hung up, killing tons of people. One of the other patients was on the phone one day and I saw him about to hang it up. I ran over and grabbed the phone from him in order to prevent him from hanging it up. We were trying to wrestle it from each other's hands until one of the nurses walked by, ripped the phone from our hands and hung it up. From then on, I thought that nurse was a terrorist because I thought his actions had caused a plane to crash, killing people.

I remember I also developed another obsession with the phones. I had missed a call from my friend Rhee one night, and I was afraid to miss another call from someone trying to reach me. I had been in my room hanging out and one of the other patients had answered the phone and told her that I was sleeping. From then on, I became super anxious about missing another phone call. So, to ensure that I didn't, I became the "secretary of the floor," so to speak. Every time the patients' phone would ring, I would come running from wherever I was and I would answer it, hoping it was for me. And if not, I would run and tell whichever patient the call was for that someone was on the phone for them.

Often throughout the week, a select group of patients were allowed to leave the floor and venture to another floor. I never knew where they were going, and I wasn't able to go due to my status. Toward the end of my stay, as my mind became more stable, I was eventually invited to go. I was super excited and referred to leaving the floor as a "field trip." I soon found out that there was a cafeteria on another floor that had a jungle theme with trees painted on the walls. Taking patients to this floor for lunch was an escape from the usual scene on the residing floor. I also remember when we got to the elevator to "go on the field trip," I crouched down low in the elevator. I thought that I was giving off too much energy, which would interfere with the operation of the elevator. I crouched down to prevent the elevator from dropping to the bottom floor. It was a pretty intense feeling.

One day I found myself in one of the lounge rooms which had a giant dry-erase board. I drew all over the board with different images of ideas that crossed my mind, such as hearts, peace signs, smiley faces, a butterfly and bumblebee, along with positive messages. I wrote "hello" in a few different languages - English, Spanish, Latin, Chinese, and Arabic. One of the other patients on the floor was Arabic and showed me how to write in Arabic including the phrase "peace be with you." The drawings and messages were all positive in nature. Examples of the types of messages I wrote included phrases like "world peace," "peace, love and happiness," and "spread love." I positioned the board so it was the first thing anyone saw when they entered the lounge.

As my stay at BryLin went on, my condition improved and the day finally arrived for me to be discharged. I was very excited to be going home and I was anxious for my parents to arrive. I lingered in front of the elevator all morning, pacing back and forth eagerly awaiting their arrival. I remember one of the nurses approaching me while I was waiting for them. I remember him making a comment about the first thing I was going to do when I left. He said the first thing I was probably going to do was smoke a cigarette. He probably thought it was an innocent comment but I was really bothered that he said this to me. I had wondered why a nurse of all people would make such a comment, especially to someone they knew had been struggling.

I remember the ride home with my parents. We were on the thru-way and were approaching a billboard sign. The billboard was of Disney's *The Little Mermaid*. I was instantly overcome with joy. Positivity flushed my brain. The billboard amplified the idea in my head that my mission had been accomplished. I had done my part in offsetting the negative vibes and I was under the impression that the world was beginning to be a better place. The lyrics "We came for salvation, we came for family, we came for all that's good that's how we walk away, we came to break the bad, we came to cheer the sad, we came to leave behind the world a better way" by The Avett Brothers resonated in my mind. Although the billboard had sparked positive feelings for me, I was feeling antsy in the backseat. I peeked into the front seat, asking my parents for a cigarette. Something I went without for about two weeks. But I had the urge and I will forever blame that nurse for putting the thought into my head. We continued our ride and approached a round-about where construction was going on. There were also some people planting flowers. Pleasantville. All I could continue to think, with a smile on my face, was that the world was a better way.

After I was discharged, one of the main focuses for my family was getting me proper treatment. Something that would help me long-term. After some research and phone calls, they found I was eligible for a program called OnTrack. OnTrack is described as "an innovative treatment program for adolescents and young adults who have recently had unusual thoughts and behaviors." This program allowed for counselors to come out to the house to meet with me if need be. And if I had episodes in the future, it would provide me with the option of staying home and possibly avoid having to go into the hospital at all. This was another reason the program appealed to my family. So, we set up my first appointment at the house.

My thoughts had become more rational than they were when I was in the hospital. However, I was still making associations. Mostly with song lyrics and people in my life. I had not completely surpassed the mania and was still waking up very early in the morning, full of energy. I would wake up around 4:30 AM-5AM and take a shower, get dressed in what I thought was the perfect colorful or meaningful outfit, and be ready to go. Downfall - not many people are awake that early in the morning. So, I spent the first few hours listening to music, watching the sunrise, writing in my notebook and pacing around the house. I was not allowed to drive due to safety concerns, of course. I would often beg to go to my favorite local diner, Teddy's, when everyone would wake up. During the day, I would spend time walking around the neighborhood with my iPod. One day I even stumbled upon a yard sale and found some things I was interested in buying. It was only a block away so I was able to walk home and get my money to return and make purchases.

A counselor came out to evaluate me shortly after my discharge from the hospital. We had an hour-long meeting. We scheduled another meeting at the house about a week later. Although my state of mind had improved since being discharged, as mentioned before, some of my irrational thoughts were still lingering. So, during these meetings I was actually under the impression that this was all a part of the movie that was being made. After a couple of meetings at the house with the counselor, we scheduled a meeting at the office where I could meet my psychiatrist.

During this period after my release from the hospital, I remember going to the cemetery with my father one day. We met my uncle and his nephew there to clean up some relatives' gravesites. I remember my uncle making a comment to me that MVP really means "Most Valuable Parent." It got me thinking and led to the following post on Facebook:

Facebook Post August 10, 2015

My uncle recently told me the true meaning of MVP: Most Valuable Parent.. Well I cherish both of my parents. My Mother Dearest always taught me—Take control of the situation, emotion…do not let the situation, emotion control you; My Father always taught me—Everything in moderation; As for me—I hope to guide Others in living life by the Golden Rule: Treat others and Mother Nature the way you would like to be treated---be RESPECTFUL... To keep it simple and not think too hard...let things come NATURALLY. A GREAT FRIEND recently bought me a sign that reads: TEACH, instruct, encourage, mentor, PRAISE, influence, GUIDE, INSPIRE. I hope to do just that..Lead by example of living RESPECTFULLY: for Self, Others and Mother Nature...with the HOPE Others will follow in my footsteps. And I firmly believe if this is accomplished.. The World would be a PEACEFUL, Bonnaroovian place: Throwing up high fives, peace signs, fist bumps, elbow bumps..Or simply a wave to fellow neighborinos. Imagine that...All the people living life in Peace...that's all John Lennon wanted....DREAMS CAN COME TRUE... as long as you...TRY TRY TRY...At least that is what my role model, Alecia Moore taught me. And in the words of another one of my role models, Ellen Degeneres, ANYYYYWAYYYY....(Crosses foot over)

KEEP CALM AND CARRY ON!

....that's my story and I'm sticking to it.

The post was evidence that my manic mindset was still present. But at that point it was somewhat under control and did seem to be diminishing.

I remember after being released from the hospital I still experienced bouts of paranoia. One day, I was at a grocery store with Rhee and I was convinced the woman standing behind us in line was taking pictures and recording me on her cell phone. Rhee kept reassuring me that she was not. I remained skeptical. On another occasion, I remember going to my grandmother's house and I feared that a white van had followed my sister and me there. Not only did I believe that it had followed us, but I believed that it was recording our conversations as well. Another time, I went out to my older sister's house and was paranoid that the neighbor adjacent to her yard was recording us. On the way back home, I was suspicious of a person in a white Lincoln that was behind us for a while. There were a lot of random instances where my paranoia was affecting me. I was still making random associations to things that stuck out to me. I remember the grain pattern on my psychiatrist's wooden door to his office was identical to the grain on a door at my sister's work. It looked like a horse's head. I found comfort in this, thinking that it meant that he was the right psychiatrist for me. I passed a street sign one day and the street was called Woodlee. I remember it reminded me of my dad, simply because he would often do home improvement projects where he would cut wood, and because he wears Lee jeans. I was constantly making these little associations with everything I crossed paths with. I remember feeling deep connections to people that had passed on. When I went to the cemetery with my father to clean off the gravesites, I remember feeling at peace and calm.

I was obsessive compulsive about random things. One afternoon, I was at my aunt's house by the pool with my cousin, Jamie. I found a toy unicorn on the ground. I set it up on the windowsill of the garage facing toward the sun. I took pH strips with different colored squares on them and placed them so they were surrounding the unicorn. It looked like colorful rays coming from the unicorn. I felt like I was guided to do this in order to create positive balance in the atmosphere. My cousin obviously had no idea what this mini-shrine meant to me. She went over and moved the unicorn. I was visibly upset and told her she cannot do that. But I never actually explained why to her.

I still found deep meaning in things. I remember going to the Erie County Fair at the end of the summer. I wanted to get my sisters a souvenir from the fair. I remember walking by vendors with jewelry and started looking around at everything. Pieces of the jewelry reminded me of my sisters. I decided to buy the pieces that had the most meaning and it did not take me long to decide which piece to buy each one of my sisters. I bought my oldest sister, Natalie, a necklace with an anchor on it because she always anchors me down and keeps me grounded by giving good advice. Like a second mother figure. I bought Carlie a musical clef symbol necklace because we shared musical interests and often made memories going to concerts together. I bought Ava a unique orange leather watch because I spent the most time with her growing up and we created many memories together throughout childhood. Buying these items with such meaning was a token of my appreciation for them being the most important people in my life who always stood by my side no matter what.

The scheduled meeting with the psychiatrist arrived. I remember being so energized that I asked if I could do crunches in the office. Both the counselor and psychiatrist said yes. So, I got down and did crunches at rapid speed. I was listening to my iPod while I tuned in and out of what my parents were talking to them about. I stumbled upon a rug tile that looked like it had a number one in the middle of it. It looked like the number one, similar to the way it appears on The Beatles album "One." This immediately made me think of The Beatles and I switched my iPod over to shuffle Beatles songs. I explained the association I made with the Beatles from the rug tile to my psychiatrist. This gave him insight into how my mind was working. From there I was scheduled to meet with my new counselor on a bi-weekly basis.

This time around I was pretty diligent with my treatment. I was always honest with my counselor and psychiatrist about how I was feeling. About things I was doing outside of counseling. One main difference this time around was the fact that I remained clean and off drugs and alcohol for months and months. In sessions I would often talk about my goals and the people in my life. One of my goals was this new idea to journal about everything I had been through with my mental health issues. So, in September of 2015 I began writing about my first episode that I experienced. This became an activity I engaged in throughout the course of my recovery.

One of the conversations I had with my psychiatrist right after I was discharged from the hospital was the option of starting to take Lithium. This would help control the mania I was having. He explained to me that there is routine bloodwork that goes along with taking the medication. He felt that it would be the best medication for me if I responded well to it. Since it was the more natural route out of all the options, I was willing to try it. So, I started with a combination of Risperidone, which is an anti-psychotic, and Lithium, a mood stabilizer. I also took Ativan as needed, which is a medication used for anxiety.

I remained on this regimen of medication for months, with tapering the doses here and there, but never fully weaning off any of the medications. Things were going well. The only two issues were the fact that I was putting weight back on and that I was still smoking cigarettes unfortunately. But again, overall, things seemed to be going well.

Shortly after my discharge, at the end of October, I learned that I was going to be a first-time aunt. I was beyond excited. So, this gave me all the more reason to make sure I remained well. For the next several months, I was faithful with my medication, abstinent from drugs and alcohol, and honest with my supports - my counselor and my psychiatrist.

Over the course of the months from winter to spring I worked on tapering off one of my medications, the Risperidone. This seemed to help curb some of the weight gain. By the time May came around, I was back to weighing 100 pounds. So, I had gained weight but had then lost it again.

June 2016 came, and I was approaching the one-year anniversary of when my boyfriend had left me. Even though this brought up some painful memories, I was also expecting the arrival of my new niece which had me happy and excited. Needless to say, I had a range of emotions that would dance around in my mind.

I remember experiencing a few instances of paranoia that June, but nothing that seemed to be concerning to me at the time. For the most part it seemed I had reached a stable period. It had been about a year since my stay at BryLin and I seemed to be going strong with my mental stability. That is until one night, when I went out with my friend, Rhee, and I started to notice that my thinking was spiraling out of control once again. That night out would be the start of another tidal wave – the start of my third episode.

"So you strike again
  Piercing my brain like a million knives
  You're like a slap in the face
  Stealing my soul and ruining my life"
-b. amber stark

Section III
HOSTAGE

SATURDAY, JUNE 25, 2016

"So, you said your name is Carlie?" asked the man I had just met at the bar. Sketched out I replied, "No." Sketched out because my sister's name is Carlie and I thought he had been sent to find her. He was just a random man at the bar who I struck up a conversation with outside. But suddenly the things he was saying were making me suspicious and paranoid. We were talking about general topics including past education and current job status. He mentioned he wanted to be a lawyer. Days earlier my sister, Carlie, had been reviewing literature about law. In what this man probably viewed as harmless small talk, I on the other hand, began to grow paranoid. I started making connections from what he was saying. Started to think he was bugged, having someone listen in on our conversation. Looking for information not about just me but also about my family. This was the first snowball of what would become yet another horrific journey. A snowballing of OCD, paranoia and delusions. The onset of my third mental breakdown.

Looking back, I now realize that days prior to this encounter at the bar, I had experienced a subtle bout of paranoia. At the time, my place of employment was located near the Peace Bridge, a bridge that connects the

U.S. to Canada. One day while I was at work, I received a phone call on my cell phone from a random number. I had missed the call and was a little skeptical of the unknown caller. I decided to call them back to find out what the call was regarding. When I called back, I said, "Hi I just had a missed call from this number. Who is this?" The man on the other end of the phone replied, "This is Steve from the Peace Bridge Apartments." I replied, "I'm sorry I think you have the wrong number," and I hung up. That phone call sparked some suspicion in me. At that point I thought I was being stalked, considering that I worked right near the Peace Bridge. I pushed the thought to the back of my head and finished off the workday. Eventually, I was able to convince myself that it was a random call and no one was stalking me. But then the conversation at the bar happened and again triggered my paranoia.

Following the night at the bar I remember other suspicious thoughts growing in my mind. I remember going to the store, Big Lots, with Rhee. As we were walking through the store, I passed by one of the young workers. I did a double-take at him, as he looked identical to the worker that often cashed me out at my local 7-11 store. I thought it was him but when I saw him, he did not greet me as if he recognized me like he often did when I would walk into 7-11. That night I was at Rhee's house and I noticed the time on the coffee maker read 4:36 AM, but the time was actually 11:36 PM. I started to wonder why she had her clock set that way. That night I went home and checked to see what time zone displayed 4:36 AM when Eastern Standard Time was 11:36 PM. I stumbled upon the fact that locations in London aligned with this time zone. Right away this struck me as odd because Rhee would often say things in a British accent. I always thought she was just trying to be funny but now I was really starting to wonder if it was something she wasn't able to always control and hide. That she would slip up and her real accent would show. I started to zoom into the map of London to the point where I could read street names. I noticed one of the street names was Prospect. I was paranoid about this, as the street Rhee was living on in Buffalo at the time was called Prospect.

As I thought about it, I wondered if Rhee had an identical twin living in London on Prospect. I thought that was the reason she had the time on her coffee maker set to 4:36 AM. That way she would know what time it was where her sibling was located in cases where she may need to call her. I started to think about the movie, *The Parent Trap*, and how the two daughters switched places. I began to think that Rhee and her twin would switch places with one another and I began to wonder if the Rhee I hung out with was always the same person. Especially since there were periods of time when her hair was curly and other periods of time when her hair was straight. This thought of the idea of "secret twins" got the wheels turning in my head. The next time I went into 7-11, I saw the cashier who days earlier I had sworn I'd seen at Big Lots. So, as he cashed me out, I asked him if he also worked at Big Lots. He informed me that he didn't but that his identical twin brother did. This immediately triggered my mind and made me very paranoid and suspicious, especially after everything with Rhee and the thoughts of her having a twin in London. This was the moment that the idea of "evil clones" started to pop into my head and suspicious thoughts started to increase.

Sunday, July 3, 2016 (a week since the night out at the bar)

My father and I went to my aunt's house to help move a new bed into the house for my cousin. I saw my cousin, Tyler, who was home visiting from Nashville, Tennessee, where he'd recently moved. But something wasn't right. I began questioning in my mind if it was really him. I had talked to him days earlier on the phone before he returned home, and he had expressed that he was very upset and not alright. But when I saw him that day, I asked, "How are you doing?" He responded, "I'm doing good." At that point, since his response did not align with what he said to me when I had last talked to him days earlier, I believed that he was a clone and that my real cousin was still in Nashville and was being tortured there. I grew terrified as I felt threatened by this concept.

I noticed things were not right. My thinking was starting to spiral out of control and I had a panic attack. I sought out help from the OnTrack hotline, the phone service provided through my counseling agency for emergency situations. The counselor on call answered and I expressed my concern of not feeling mentally okay. I needed to talk to my psychiatrist. I was afraid to say too much over the phone. The counselor said he would try to get in contact with my psychiatrist for me. But seeing that it was a holiday weekend he was not sure if he would be able to reach my psychiatrist right away. It turned out my psychiatrist was out of town visiting family. I was really upset with how the counselor handled my concerns. Mainly because I asked him what I should do and he didn't provide much further support or guidance on what I should do in the meantime. Instead, he just asked back, "What do you think you should do?" That upset me because the thoughts seemed to be getting rapidly worse and I wasn't sure I would be able to make it through until my psychiatrist returned. I was worried for what was to come.

Monday, July 4, 2016

Paranoia had grown strong. I stayed home from my cousin's annual 4th of July party. I was freaking out too much inside to go. I refused to say too much to anyone. My mother and I went to my Aunt Teresa's house for a little while instead. Scenarios were whirling like a tornado in my mind. My aunt mentioned that my cousin had friends over swimming the night before. With my paranoia convincing me that my cousin and aunt were clones, I was under the impression that they were evil. I thought that my cousin's clone and his friends had drowned people that they had captured in their pool the night before. That would explain the bag of random sunglasses that my aunt had on her kitchen table. I looked into the bag of sunglasses in disbelief, thinking that they belonged to the people who had been drowned by my cousin's clone and his friends. As I peeked into the bag, I remember my aunt's clone asking me if I needed a pair of sunglasses. I looked at her terrified, thinking she was trying to frame me for murder.

We ventured outside to sit by the pool. I looked toward the window of the garage. The reflection in the window resembled the screen of a small television. I was frightened, suddenly struck by the thought that there was a terrorist in the garage. He was watching our every move while broadcasting news stories on this so-called T.V. The stories were all related to different terrorist attacks. I turned to the left towards my sister Ava's house, who lived next door to my aunt. I noticed through the window her husband sitting on the back screened-in patio with his back towards me. He had his arms raised up and his hands resting on the back of his head. All I could think of was that he was being held hostage by terrorists at gunpoint. He was a veteran and it was the 4th of July. I thought he was being targeted. My heart began to race. I glanced back at the phantom T.V. in the garage window. Though I was panicking on the inside, I was trying to remain outwardly calm in order to avoid setting off the terrorists. I told my mother I wanted to go home.

Things were getting worse and I was flooded with irrational thoughts. Similar to the second episode, I do not remember the exact order of the following thoughts. I just recall having them. Therefore, most of the thoughts will be listed in a random order of occurrence. The ideas aren't linear, which is a conscious style choice. The paragraphs jump from thought to thought without much order to them, which as fair warning, can be jarring. I did this to give insight as to what it's like inside the mind of someone with mania and paranoia. So, reading the following passages may be overwhelming and disorienting, which is often how it feels to someone experiencing these thoughts.

Fourth of July night there were a lot of fireworks going off. I was never sure if what I was hearing was worrisome or not. At times, I was convinced I was hearing rounds of gunshots. My mind was directed toward the idea of clones. The clones were invading South Buffalo, like the zombies on the T.V. show, "The Walking Dead." My family had to keep convincing me it was just fireworks. Feeling terrified, I paced through the house. I noticed the statue of the Virgin Mary we have set up in the house. Seeing it made me think I should pray. I retrieved my glow in the dark rosary from my bedroom. It was the same rosary I held close following my episode in 2015. I paced the downstairs of my house through the back room to the dining room to the living room, back and forth, praying. I repeatedly recited the "Glory Be," the "Lord's Prayer," and the "Hail Mary." I dedicated my prayers to the poor, the starving, perseverance, prosperity and to overall world peace. As I paced and prayed, I focused in on the statue of Mary as I passed by her. I thought of the song "Let It Be" by the Beatles. Specifically, the lyrics "When I find myself in times of trouble Mother Mary comes to me, speaking words of wisdom let it be. And in my hour of darkness, she is standing right in front of me, speaking words of wisdom let it be."

I ventured to the porch for a cigarette. I heard a windchime from the neighboring house. I also noticed the motion light on the garage across the street turn on. I was overwhelmed with paranoia due to the suspicion that these two stimuli created within me. I thought that the chime was a signal notifying the clones that I was on the porch so that they could drive by and shoot me. As I sat in the chair on the porch, the motion light appeared to get brighter. I was under the impression that the light was getting brighter to help the clones focus in on me. I took one last drag of my cigarette and I rushed inside.

That night I was lying in bed. I woke up to voices outside the window at 3:00 in the morning. I peeked out of the blinds to see three young boys with backpacks walking down the middle of the street. I was terrified. I thought that they were a part of the "Irish Mafia Clones," another delusion that suddenly formed in my head. With South Buffalo being a predominantly Irish heritage neighborhood, and after I'd been hearing "gunshots" all night, in my mind I concluded that a war had begun between the Irish residents and the clones of the Irish residents.

I remember being at 7-11 earlier that day buying cigarettes. I noticed a couple in the store that I knew. They were the parents of a boy who I had attended grammar school with when I was younger. But they didn't seem to make eye contact with me. And they had drawn looks on their faces. I was put off, thinking that I had done something wrong. Why didn't they say hello? But then a thought clicked in my head: any person that came into contact with me, if I knew the person, they would die. If they showed that they knew me in any way, if I said that I recognized them or if I mentioned that they looked like someone else I knew, or like a celebrity, then they would be targeted by the bad guys. With this in mind, every time I heard a "gunshot," I was under the impression that the clones had killed a hostage that I knew. I believed that they had acquired random homes throughout South Buffalo, where they would imprison people, torture them and eventually kill them. I believed they purposely chose to carry out their mission during July to cover up the sounds of gunshots and lead people to believe they were fireworks. I also remember reading an article a few weeks prior about the movie *The Purge*, which had a plot that involved a one-night-a-year exemption that allowed people to go on crime and murder sprees without repercussions. Recalling this article fed into my fear, as I thought something similar may be going on in our neighborhood. As terrified as I was, I knew I had to remain calm. Making the wrong move would just contribute to the chaos. And saying anything to anyone was out of the question.

I remember going to have a cigarette on my back deck. I took a drag and heard voices. They sounded like they were coming from the garage. I could not make out what was being said but I thought they were saying things along the lines of me being a bad person and I needed to let them out of the garage. The voices were muffled and there were multiple voices at once. So, it was hard to tell exactly what they were saying. I put my cigarette out and I went back inside. I was scared. At that point I thought that my family might have been evil clones and not their true selves. And that they were keeping people in the garage that they would later kill. I had seen a box of garbage bags in my dad's truck earlier that day. I thought that they were used for the dead bodies. I went into the living room. My mother and father were in the kitchen having a conversation. I thought I heard my mother say to my father, "we need to get rid of Carlie's body. It is going to start to smell." I thought she was referring to my sister Carlie being dead. And I thought that the "Carlie" I saw from that point on was really a clone.

It was about 5:30 in the morning one day and I was getting ready to go have a cigarette on the porch. I noticed my neighbor backing his truck into my driveway and I froze in my steps. Suspicion overcame me. I wondered what he was doing. Why so early? What was he hiding? He backed the truck into our driveway really far, to the point where I could no longer see his truck bed from the porch doorway. I figured he was putting bags of dead bodies from my garage on his truck bed to dispose of them. The truck pulled out and behind it walked a man in a green and black checkered flannel. From behind he resembled Steven Avery from the documentary *Making a Murderer*. I began to think it was him and that he was framing my family for murder. That he was working with the clones of my family in a murder operation ring in South Buffalo. I waited until the coast seemed clear to go out on the porch. Anxiety-ridden, I went out to the porch. The neighbor's wind chime sounded. I was sitting on the porch chair and I noticed a bird on the front lawn. I began to think that the eye of the bird was really a camera and that the bird was recording me. Of course, for the bad guys. I was afraid to make eye contact with it for more than a couple seconds. I believed that making eye contact with the bird enabled it to access thoughts and memories from my mind. This concept of the birds being cameras haunted me every time I went out on the porch and saw them. Whenever I would walk out of the house, I would hear a crow caw. Similar to the wind chimes, I believed the crow was cawing to alert the bad guys that I was out in public. Therefore, a lot of the ideas and beliefs flooding my mind made it difficult to leave the house. I felt taunted every time and straight-up scared.

The couch in our back room was a love seat that reclined with a footrest. I noticed that when my dad would get off the couch, he would never fully put the foot rest down. He would just push it enough for him to get off the couch. He would even leave it up when he left the house. I thought he was doing this intentionally because if he closed it, there would be an explosion.

There was a slight breeze one day as I sat on our front porch. I became distracted by the waving of the American Flag on our house. I noticed that it was pretty beat up and in rough shape with frayed and ripped edges. I thought we needed to replace it sooner than later, as it is disrespectful to our country to fly a torn-up flag. I became paranoid about what other people would think of my family for showing such disrespect. I began looking around at the other neighbors' flags. I noticed one of our neighbors had a Boston Red Sox flag. My mindset was similar to my first episode where certain teams exhibited positive energy and others negative energy. In this case, the Red Sox were bad simply because I remember my grandfather and grandmother being Yankees fans growing up. Therefore, I believed the person in the house with the Red Sox flag was a clone and that it was one of the houses where they kept the South Buffalo prisoners.

I was also convinced that there were bad guys under our deck in the backyard. The way the deck was constructed, there were two pieces of wood layered on top of each other, forming a wall. Between the two pieces of wood was a space. I thought that the bad guys would hide under the deck and shoot a laser beam through the space to try and harm us. My dad suffers from Gout, and I began to think that these lasers were the cause. He would sit on the couch with his feet reclined on the footrest, and I believed that the bad guys would shoot a laser beam at his ankles. This would later aggravate his Gout and cause him pain, making it hard for him to walk.

Another trip to the back deck for a cigarette. I noticed the rug underneath the grill was all black as if it were burned. The grill must have been left on. The bad guys did it. They had the ability to control our thoughts and actions if we did not protect ourselves. Negative feelings allowed for the bad guys to control us even more. So, if someone was in a bad mood, then the bad guys could control how that person behaved; what they did, what they said and what they thought. Not just me. Everyone. Therefore, I thought that there must have been a moment when whoever was using the grill became weak and vulnerable and the bad guys controlled their thoughts, making them forget to turn the grill off. Because the bad guys wanted the house to burn down.

One day as I looked out of my second story bedroom window, I noticed that the patio umbrella was opened on our back deck. I was looking down at it and the top of the umbrella reminded me of Pinocchio. The tip of the umbrella resembled his lying nose. My mind had simultaneously shifted to another Disney themed notion, and the thought that flashed through my mind was that I was a "lost boy". A "lost boy" among a sea of clones.

My sister Carlie, or her clone rather, was sitting on the back deck. I went out there to have a cigarette. I was focused on her shirt. It was a red t-shirt with a dog on it. It said, "Unleashed Excitement." I saw this message as a sign, and I thought it meant that the bad guys were going to try to get my dogs to fight each other, or more often, other dogs. My dogs are microchipped, so I thought they were able to be controlled through their microchips by the bad guys. Therefore, I thought the bad guys were always making them bark in the house or go crazy when we were on walks and would pass other dogs on the street. My younger dog would also constantly chase his tail. I thought he was being controlled to do that through the microchip.

My older dog had a really big belly. She would lie on the floor and I would be worried she was going to explode because I thought she had a bomb in her stomach. I thought she was linked to my dad because my dad has a hernia and it juts out of his stomach. It seemed to appear bigger to me than usual. I was under the impression that the bomb in his stomach was getting bigger meaning that it could explode at any moment. I thought that it was important to keep both my dog and my dad calm or it could trigger the bomb to go off in their stomachs.

I believed there was a man in the basement. He would control the temperature of the house. Common sense was not really in the cards for me, considering my thoughts were mostly irrational. So, the fact that it was summer was never the reason as to why the house was so hot. Instead, it was the man in the basement making it that way. The heat would agitate me and I would run my head under cold water in the kitchen sink to cool off. Or I would open the freezer door and stand in the freezer for a few minutes.

There was a thick orange rope that we would hook my dog to when he would go outside. To me it was a directive from the man in the basement to hook him up to it. And I thought it was actually a gas line. I was under the impression that if my dog acted too wild and pulled too hard on the rope, the gas line would bust, gas would leak out and there would be an explosion. So, I would freak out on the inside when the rope would get kinked or tangled. I would constantly fix it so it was straight.

I was afraid to go upstairs alone at first and then eventually at all because I thought that there was an evil person lurking up there. This was an issue considering the shower was upstairs. So, I started to wash my hair in the kitchen sink. I would also wash my feet too. Another thing I thought the man in the basement was controlling was the temperature of the water from the kitchen faucet. When you would turn the water on it would come out scalding hot. Even if you turned on the cold water, it would still come out hot at first before turning cold. So, it was very easy to burn yourself. I thought the man in the basement was intentionally trying to hurt us or test our ability to remember to be careful.

The man in the basement would also track my every move. If I was in bare feet, he could track me. I believed he created a system that used coils embedded throughout the floor of the downstairs and in the ceiling of the basement. The coils would absorb temperature from bare feet. Then the system would deliver the location of the feet to a computer that displayed a map of the house. Infrared markers on the map displayed on the computer screen would inform the man in the basement of my location. To avoid him being able to track me, I always wore sandals and slippers throughout the house. I figured he was not able to trace the temperature of my feet this way.

The door to our front porch has a metal stopper to adjust the door to keep it opened. I believed that if the metal tab was pushed over to the other side to prop the door open, touching the other piece of metal, a signal would be sent to the man in the basement. He would then trigger a control that would set off a ticking time bomb. To stop the time bomb I believed you had to unprop the door so that the metal pieces were not touching. Therefore, I was constantly unpropping the door when my family would open it. I would use a pillow to prop the door instead. I could not tell my family why though, or we would be killed.

There is also a sliding lock on the outside of our basement door. If it is locked, you are not able to get up from the basement. I believed that the man in the basement had snuck into the house to rob us and murder my family but had gotten stuck in the basement. I spent days thinking he was down there. I was terrified over the concept. I would constantly walk past the basement and lock the door. As soon as someone would open it, I would be right behind them to close and lock it back up. I did not want the man to come out. I believed it was like the concept of vampires. They won't enter your territory unless you invite them in. If the door was left opened it would give the man the impression that he was invited into our space. One day, I remember being in the kitchen, which is right near the basement door. My dog was lying in front of the basement door. I heard someone whisper. I turned quickly toward the voice which sounded like it was coming from the basement. I believed the man was trying to get my dog's attention to roll over and knock open the door so that he could get out and harm me. Another time, when I was in the kitchen wetting my hair, I heard an evil whistle come from the basement door. Almost like a prelude letting me know he was about to kill me.

I started to think that cars that were driving by our house were "speaking to me" when I was on the front porch smoking. I thought they were sending me signals about what I should do. I would be on the porch smoking a cigarette, pacing back and forth. A car would drive by slowly and that would indicate that I could take my time with smoking my cigarette. But if a car drove by quickly, it would mean that I needed to hurry up and get back in the house. Slow cars could also mean that I needed to slow my thoughts and behavior down. That if I moved too quickly, disaster would ensue. These thought processes would occur every time I would go on the porch. Most of the time I had to hurry up and smoke my cigarette and get back inside to prevent the guy in the basement from blowing my mother's oxygen machine up. At one point I thought a movie was being filmed.

I would see old-fashioned cars drive by and think they were purposely planted for the movie. People walking by the house were also purposely planted.

There was a girl walking by the house one day. I was convinced she was a girl I worked with that had cut her hair short. She had her phone in her hand when she walked by. I believed she was playing "Pokémon Go" on her phone. My idea of "Pokémon Go" was that the characters in the game represented people in the real world. Certain characters would provide a certain number of points. If you had the game up while walking down the street, the game would capture surrounding people whom would be translated into the game. And if you identified the character's location, you would get the points that the character represented. Since I seemed to be a target for the bad guys, I felt that I was a character that provided a lot of points. When the girl walked by with her phone up, she looked towards me. I thought she had figured out that my Pokémon character was wanted by the bad guys and that revealing my location would give her a lot of points. Terrified, I ran into the house.

I would have horrible anxious thoughts about people in my family or about anyone in my life, really. About bad things happening to them. One thing I always worried about was that people were going to try and light my mother's oxygen machine on fire. Ultimately, I believed the man in the basement would be the one to do it. That's when the song lyrics, "I can't feel my face when I'm with you," from the song "Can't Feel My Face" by The Weeknd, popped into my head. I imagined that my actions, or lack thereof, would lead to the man in the basement lighting the hose to the machine with a lighter. The fire would travel to my mother's face and burn it off. Really, I pictured an explosion going off in her face. It would terrify me. This horrific thought would cycle through my mind on a daily basis.

We had three dogs in the house. Two were mine and one was my sister's. Often times they would lie on the ground next to each other in a straight line. This placement tipped off a warning to me. The three dogs lying in a line would create negative energy. So, I was constantly making sure that when they were lounging together that they didn't form a line. I would move one of the dogs out of placement if they were lined up. Again, I thought this created negative energy and that it would create an atmosphere where bad things would happen.

The number of people in a room at one time also became a concern of mine. Only five people were allowed in a room at one time. If there were more than five people, things would be unbalanced and negative energy would be created around the house and the world. If there were five people already in a room I would not go in there. If there were more, I would try to call someone out of the room to balance it.

I remember going to 7-11 one night and seeing that the cashier had a swastika on his shirt. I was freaked out, as I thought of the evil and the torture committed by the Nazi's. He cashed me out and gave me my change that equaled $1.38. As he handed me the change he remarked, "138, that's a good number." I immediately wondered what he meant by that and started creating scenarios in my mind. I came to the conclusion that on July 11th (7-11, because of the store) at 1:38 (my change amount) AM or PM, clones were going to come to my home and try to kill me. Or, if they weren't going to kill me, something bad was going to happen.

I made note of the cars parked on the street. I noticed that three of the vehicles on the street were the same kind of cars that were owned by three of my family members. A silver car, a blue truck and a red truck. I thought that this was done purposely. Purposely to confuse the bad guys, and keep them from knowing when my family was at the house or not. The more people that were at the house, the less likely they would be to try to attack me. I thought the similar vehicles would be parked on the street if my family was not home in order to make it seem like they were at the house.

Vehicles on the road had either the old New York State license plates, which were white, or the new New York State license plates, which were yellow. I started to become sketched out by the difference. I began creating an idea in my head attaching a reason to why people had the different styles of license plates. I immediately went outside to see which style my family had on the cars. We all had white plates. Just then I believed that humans had white plates and clones had yellow plates. After that I started questioning all the people that had cars with a yellow license plate.

I took my dogs out with my dad one night for a short walk down the street. As we were headed back to the house, I noticed a car in my neighbor's driveway. As we got closer, I could hear a baby crying through the car window. I was concerned. I thought that they had abducted my newborn niece. I literally walked to the front of their car as they were pulling out of the driveway and stared them down. I memorized the license plate so that I could have one of my friends, who is a police officer, run the plate and track them down. We had watched the movie *Finding Dory* earlier that week and I thought that this was the real-life version of "Finding Dory," but instead we needed to find my niece. I remember hearing a train later that night. *The Girl on the Train* was another popular movie at the time. I started to make a connection with the movie title and the notion that I thought my niece was abducted. I believed that my real niece was on the train. This scenario of my niece being abducted and being on the train gave the movie title a new meaning to me now. I started to believe that movie titles were actually predictions about my life.

I began to wonder if everyone that surrounded me was a clone. I had been switching back and forth between whether or not certain members of my family and friends were clones. One second, I would decide that they were, and the next, they weren't. I had an inkling that my one sister was a clone and that she had given my niece to my neighbors in the car. In turn they gave my sister a clone of the baby. I had the notion in my head that it took three weeks for a clone to be created. Seeing that it had been three weeks since my niece had been born, I figured that her clone was now full-grown to her actual size. I also started to reflect back on my past and the fact that I had been at the hospital for three weeks during my stay for my first episode. I started to wonder if all of my family members were really clones. That my real family had been abducted and the clones were created while I was staying at the hospital during my first episode. Therefore, by the time I got out of the hospital, everyone in my family had been replaced by clones. I started to get scared and feel alone. "Where is my real family and who are these clones? What do they want with me? What did they do to my family?" Then I started to create more scenarios. My family was being tortured and enslaved up at ECMC, the first hospital I stayed at. I imagined this had been going on for the past three years. Thinking they were tortured, starved and physically beaten. I imagined them with blind-folds, their hands tied behind their back with no clothes on, emaciated with welts, bruises, and scars all over their bodies. The only one that wasn't physically beaten was my father. He was mentally beaten. I thought that he was constantly tied to a chair and forced to watch my mother and my sisters be physically and sexually abused. I believed the clone of my father was ordering all of this to happen. I remember hearing the song "Start Me Up" by The Rolling Stones and focusing on the lyrics from the song, "You make a grown man cry-y-y." Images of my real father witnessing the abuse and crying because of it flooded my mind. My real father was allowed to come home every 48 hours. But only allowed to stay for 24 hours. And during that time, he had to put in long hours of manual labor. I remember he brought steak home for dinner one night. He seasoned the steak and ate quietly at the table. I thought this was a directive from the father clone. I went to taste my steak. I couldn't eat it. It tasted funny to me. In hindsight, I think that odd taste was a symptom I was experiencing just like during my first episode. I do not think there was anything wrong with the steak. But at the time I thought the seasoning was poison and that the father clone had directed my father to put the seasoning on the steak.

There were also cases of bottled water at our house that triggered my paranoia. The case of Nestle PureLife water had labels on the bottles that included the number 150 inside a circle, to commemorate the company's 150th anniversary. Labels often had meaning to me. In this case, I believed that the water was tainted because of the "150" label. I believed that if I drank the water my heart rate would increase to 150 and I would have a heart attack. The other case of water was the brand "Big Win." I would always drink this, as I thought the name suggested that it was safer. I would drink water constantly throughout the day as I thought it was necessary since I was on Lithium and I would get overheated easily. I was constantly refilling the refrigerator with bottles throughout the day.

One day I was on the front porch and I noticed the placement of an empty bottle of "Big Win" water. It was placed in front of the lamp on the table, which I perceived as being an intentional placement. I thought it was to prevent the bad guys from shooting the lightbulb to the lamp and breaking it. I thought someone in my family had placed the water bottle in front of the lamp subconsciously to prevent the lamp from being targeted and to protect me. I started to think that my left eye would glow in the dark. And when I was on the porch at night, I would turn the lamp on so my eye would not glow and the bad guys could not identify that it was me on the porch. I left the "Big Win" water bottle there for days. I would occasionally think about the water bottle being there. Once again, I entertained the idea that, similar to the second episode I had, my life was really a movie being recorded. I started to think that at the end of everything that was going on, if I could overcome the evil forces, it would be considered "the big win." So, I thought it was possible that the last scene of the movie would be video footage of me standing on the porch smoking a cigarette, with the "Big Win" water bottle in the background, and the camera would zoom in on the water bottle as the final shot. Furthermore, the movie would be called "The Big Win."

Since I was afraid to go upstairs because I thought someone was up there, I would do laundry and sort it out on the kitchen table. I would leave my folded laundry in piles on the table for the course of my episode. I remember having my sister go upstairs to get me clothes from my room if there was something in particular that I needed. She was brave enough. I also had the lingering thought in my head that the man in the basement had a plan to attack me. I would wear certain items of clothing that I thought protected me. Similar to my first two episodes, I eventually got to the point where I thought it was dangerous to wear clothing with writing on it. If there was a sports player's name on my clothes, I was afraid that they would be in harm's way. If there was a certain team name on the clothes, like the Bills, Sabres, or Blackhawks, I thought that the players on the team and their families would get bad luck and be harmed. So, I got to the point where I would wear only solid colors and shirts with no writing or images on them.

I used to lay on the chair in our living room. Behind the chair is a staircase to the upstairs. I thought that the person upstairs was going to try and shoot me from the landing of the staircase. Because I took Lithium, I believed that the bullets would be able to target me easier. I thought Lithium attracted the metal/lead from the bullets. There was a blanket that had a teddy bear on it. I believed that this blanket had protective properties like a shield. I would lay under this blanket in order to prevent the bullets from striking me. Similar to the person upstairs, I also thought that the man in the basement was trying to harm me by shooting harmful lasers at me through the bottom of the couch when I would sit on it. Therefore, I would cover the couch with a tan blanket, which I also believed to have protective properties, before sitting or lying on the couch. The blanket would prevent the man from detecting me on the couch and prevent him from being able to shoot the harmful lasers at me.

Eventually, I mustered up the courage to go upstairs again. I made my sisters walk me through each room to see if there was anyone in there. Rest assured my suspicions were debunked. And the coast was clear. However, I was still afraid to shower alone. So, I would have one of my sisters sit in the bathroom while I showered as quickly as I could of course. And with music. I would shout for them to play music and to turn it up louder.

I was afraid that the man in the basement was planning to tamper with my medicine. I wasn't sure whether he was going to do it himself, or if he was going to order someone else to break in and do it. So, I was protective of my medicine and where I kept it. I had it in my mind that he and his accomplices were not able to approach wooden cupboards. So, I thought that anything that I put inside our wooden cupboards or wooden drawers was safe.

I used to smoke Marlboro Ultra Lights, which come in a silver pack. My sister and cousin used to smoke "Marlboro Golds," which come in a gold pack. I started to think that clones smoked Marlboro Golds. So, I became suspicious of anyone that smoked Marlboro Golds, including my sister and my cousin. I started to question things that they would say to me or things they would do.

Another paranoid thought that revisited me from my previous episode was an issue I had with my peacock sneakers. Again, I thought they had a bomb linked to them. So, like my episode in 2015, I took the peacock sneakers and put them in a paper bag. I rolled the bag closed and put the bag out by the shed as quickly as I could. I wanted nothing to do with the sneakers. They freaked me out.

I believed that mirrors were recording devices where I was being watched. Every mirror in the house was a way for the bad guys to spy on me. I thought they were using the mirror as a way to access information to use against me. I remember feeling insecure about getting out of the shower because of the mirrors in the bathroom. I also remember when I finally started sleeping in my own room upstairs again there was a mirror in there. I would lie in bed at night freaked out at the idea that I was being watched while I was asleep. Therefore, I took a blanket and covered the mirror.

I remember watching T.V. one day and there was a sporting event on. During the intermission there was a marching band. One of the band-members looked like she was possessed. The way she shifted her head and glared her eyes. It was terrifying. That same day I went on Facebook and saw one of my friend's posts. It was a video of the same girl from the band with a strange, possessed look on her face. I took her body language and facial expressions as a threat and as a message that the enemy was coming for me. I also watched the news that day. There was a story involving the Buffalo Police, and they showed footage of officers standing in the street. I just remember seeing one of the officers on the broadcast standing in the street with this stern look on his face. It was as if he was looking right at me through the T.V. screen. I happened to know the officer as he was a relative of one of my childhood friends. The thing that stood out the most was the fact that he had piercing blue eyes. And he looked very mad. It was a terrifying look. The possessed bandmember also had piercing blue eyes. This similar feature among the two, along with their stern looks, made me think that they were clones from the same team; my enemies' team. The idea of the "South Buffalo War" that I had imagined before seemed to be even more real at this point.

My next-door neighbors had a lamp post in their backyard. I started to notice that it was always on, every day and every night. It never went off. I thought that it signified that the boys who lived next door were in the garage watching my family and making plans to attack my family. They would use computers and create algorithms that would generate negative energy to our household which would cause problems for my family and me. I would often see the boys go in the garage with a group of friends right at dusk, which only increased my suspicions.

My cousin had lost her cell phone and needed to borrow my mom's phone until she got a new one. She had her contacts added to my mom's phone while she used it. Eventually she gave the phone back. I remember using my mom's phone one day and seeing the contacts that had been added. I instantly got freaked out and wondered why my cousin would have such famous people in her phone. I remember one of the names in the phone being Ellen. I immediately thought it was Ellen Degeneres' number. I thought I was being watched and would get in trouble for looking at the phone so I would slam it shut and hide it away. I got to thinking that I was not supposed to have access to all of these celebrities' phone numbers. That my cousin was a clone and had stolen the phone with the celebrities' information in it. I was under the impression that some of the celebrities were out to find the phone and get it back to prevent their personal information from being shared with anyone. I was terrified and just wanted to give the phone back. I thought that the phone had a tracking device on it and they were able to trace it to my house. So, I devised a plan that I would leave the phone in a purse by the door so that they would come into the house and grab it while my family and I were asleep at night.

The purse I decided to use was one a coworker had given to me as a gift. I had been grateful for the gift at first. But when everything started to get out of control in my mind, I started to think that the purse had a tracking device in it. I suddenly didn't want the purse anymore. So, I grabbed the purse, leaving all the money that was inside of it because I thought that the celebrities would be expecting it as ransom money. Then I put the celebrity cellphone in the purse, along with the money, and placed it by the door. Every night I would expect that they would come retrieve it. But each morning, I would wake up to see the purse still there. Being confused, I left it there. It remained by the door throughout my episode until my thoughts cleared up and I was thinking rationally again.

I recently had purchased a new Champion baseball cap that was gray and pink. I remember seeing my neighbor out in front of the house as she was walking to her car. She was wearing a pair of gray shorts with pink trim on them. Just like my hat. As she passed by me, she grabbed her purse and shook it, jingling her keys. I thought that gesture of her jingling her keys was her tipping off a shooter to shoot me. I hurried to get inside.

Taking my dogs out to go to for a walk always seemed very calculated. I'd get out to the front yard and by the time I got there my mom would be sitting on the porch. As if she was watching to make sure everything went smoothly. My dad, the dogs and I would walk down our street to the same driveway every time and then cross the street. And then we would walk back. It was key to not see any other dogs on the street because this would rile my dogs up. Whenever we would see another dog on the street, I thought it was the clones trying to get my dogs into a fight. My dogs would go crazy and I thought the bad guys were controlling them through their microchips.

I believed that my dogs had to be cared for properly otherwise they would be taken away from me and bad things would happen in the world. I was constantly filling their water dish so it was always full and fresh. I was constantly making sure they were fed and taken out to go to the bathroom at the same time every day. I was under the impression that if I slipped up in any way, the enemies would send a truck to get the dogs. Even picking up the dog poop on our walks was important. And if I didn't or if I missed any, then bad things would happen. I even remember going to the store with my father one day. On our way back, as we were driving down our street, we passed by a strange looking white van with a red decal on it. I immediately panicked inside thinking they had just taken my dogs from my house.

I remember walking the dogs one night and we got to the part of the street where we would usually turn around. As we were crossing the street my dad pointed to the house in front of us and said, "check out that window at the top, isn't it pretty neat?" He was referring to the window's unique shape. I was instantly terrified and told my dad to stop pointing. I thought someone was watching from the window. I thought it was one of the designated houses that the clones were using to torture people. In this case, I thought my sister was in there being tortured. I thought this because the number on the house was the same as the number of the public school my sister worked at.

I started focusing in on minute details around the house. I started to spot "booby traps" around the house. The fabric of the chair in the living room had started to come off. As a result, the thick staples on the fabric were being exposed. I noticed this one day and thought that the man in the basement was using negative energy to make the fabric turn out. It was easy to cut yourself on the staples that were exposed. I would constantly turn the fabric inward to prevent anyone from being able to get cut.

On the front porch we have wicker furniture. I noticed that part of the braided wood was warped and a sharp piece of the wood was poking out. I thought this was another way the man in the basement was using negative energy to set a booby trap for someone to get hurt.

The rug on the front porch kept curling and kinking up on the one side. I thought the man in the basement was causing the rug to get kinked. Anyone passing over it needed to be mindful not to trip and fall. I was always concerned about my mom tripping over the kinked rug. I would constantly straighten it out but it would always kink back up again. And in my mind, I would always blame the man in the basement.

My sisters, my mother, my Aunt Marie, and I were all playing a game called Sequence on the front porch one day. My thoughts were instantly influenced by the moves that my family members were making in the game. We were divided into teams of two, and one team used green chips and the other team used red chips. I thought that the colors of the chips indicated whether I should "stop" or "go." Red would mean to stop and green would mean to go. These weren't the actual rules of the game, but instead related to the irrational thoughts I was having at the time. The board game consisted of a deck of cards arranged in a certain order. As my sisters, mom and aunt would choose certain cards to place their chips on, I would focus in on which card they chose along with the chip color. I believed that each specific move they made had meaning and that they were secretively trying to tell me something. Whether the card they chose to lay down on was red or black; a club, diamond, spade, or heart; as well as the number or letter of the card; each of these things played a role into my thoughts. I would also take things from the conversations they were having and tie them into my reasoning. I would flip-flop between thinking one person was a clone and the other wasn't. Even though they seemed to be enjoying themselves, the game for me was very stressful.

As we were playing, my relatives who lived down the street were walking past the house and decided to stop in and see us. When they came into the house my dogs were barking at them, specifically at my cousin's girlfriend. This was a red flag to me and made me suspicious of her. I started to think she was on the bad team in the "South Buffalo War." I started feeding into my thoughts, going as far as thinking that she was a serial killer. And now she had been "invited" into our house, so I believed that meant that she could now enter whenever she wanted to. I was under the impression that she was going to plot to kill my family.

During my episode I thought that if someone repeated something three times or more that bad things would happen. If I was ever talking to someone and they asked me to repeat what I had said a third time, I would either reword the way I said it or I would just say nevermind. That same day while we were on the porch, another one of my cousins pulled up in front of the house. He was still in the street but there weren't any cars coming. He rolled his window down and my Aunt Marie started talking to him. She asked him, "Where are you going?" He responded, "What?" and she repeated herself. Again, he had trouble hearing her and responded, "What?" My aunt then, for a third time, said "Where are you going?" My cousin then said, "Oh, shit!" and pulled away quickly. I knew right then that because my aunt had repeated herself three times that it was not a good situation. And I thought that my cousin had said, "Oh, shit!" because he realized my aunt had repeated herself three times. This just reinforced the notion I had of repeating things three times. In hindsight, I realize that he had said "oh shit" because he was blocking traffic from passing through on the street and had to move his car out of the way, not because she had repeated herself.

As I was pacing on the porch, I came across a sharp knife on one of the shelves. I grabbed it, wondering why it was there. When I grabbed it, the knife was all sticky. I immediately thought that the knife was planted evidence from the murders in our garage. I thought that the real killers, the clones, had planted the knife and made it sticky so that my fingerprints would stick to the knife better. I was immediately scared, thinking that I was screwed and I put the knife back. I remember thinking about it for days. Every time I would go on the porch, I would see it and just think that I was going to be arrested for a murder I did not commit. I would constantly think of ways to tell the police it really was not me. Eventually when my irrational thoughts subsided, I asked my dad why it was out there. He told me it was there in the case of a fire so that we could cut our way out of the screen if we needed to escape. Needless to say, this gave me peace of mind.

I remember being afraid to charge my phone. I thought the electrical currents were going to cause an explosion. So, to save my battery for emergencies I would shut my phone off. I also had the same thought about my phone being on in general. That it was going to cause an explosion if I used it. So, I would only charge it for a few minutes if I needed to. And I would just turn it on to see text messages I'd received and would quickly shut it off after I read them.

One day my two sisters, my aunt, my mom, my niece and my sister's best friend were going shopping for a wedding dress in Rochester, NY for my sister's wedding. It was an hour or so away from home. I decided to go along for the trip. I got in the car and right from the beginning I was super anxious. As the car ride continued, I started to question the clones in the car. I came to the conclusion that my older sister, Natalie, was the only one that was not a clone. As we got to Rochester, we were driving on the highway. I started to imagine the end of the highway leading to a cliff where we were going to fall off. Like the end of the Earth. My sister had her navigation on and Siri was telling her to take the next exit. And I could have sworn that at the exit, Siri said to make a left. But my sister made a right. I started to think we were being tricked, but that my sister knew how to trump the tricks so we wouldn't fall off the Earth. She knew to do the opposite of what Siri was telling us to do. We were driving through town and I noticed some graffiti on a public trash can on the sidewalk. It said "The world is flat." This freaked me out, as it confirmed the idea of the highway ending at a cliff. At this point, I was in desperate need of a cigarette. We finally got to the bridal shop and went inside. I lasted not even five minutes before I headed outside with my aunt to have a cigarette. I was not speaking much at all. I may have just mentioned that I needed water. As I was smoking, I noticed a gas station a block and a half away. I started to walk toward the gas station to find out that it wasn't even there and it was just a sign with an empty lot. I felt like I was trapped in a bad dream. After the shop we drove around to find a place to eat. They decided they wanted to eat at a restaurant called Uno. Of course, this was suspicious to me. At this point I thought they were trying to tell me that I was the only "one," considering the restaurant was called Uno. That I was the only real one and they were all clones. From there I freaked out even more on the inside and dreaded the hour-long ride home with these clones. One of the things I was certain I should not do was let them know that I knew they were clones. Otherwise, they would hurt my real family members.

I remember going home that night and sitting on the couch with my mother, who I obviously thought was a clone. I had been overwhelmed with emotion and exhaustion of constantly having to deal with all these frightening scenarios swirling around my head. And without giving away too much of what I had been thinking about lately I made a concerning comment. I told her I did not think I could go on like this any longer. She reached her hand out to me and placed it on my shoulder and started to cry. She told me not to say that and that she would not know what to do without me. I started to flip back to thinking she was my real mother and not a clone because of her reaction. That she was now the only one I could trust.

Prior to the onset of my episode, my sister, Ava, had asked if I'd be interested in joining in on a Harry Potter Escape Room with her and some other friends and family members. I had told her that I wanted to go when we initially talked about it. The day of the event came and everyone met at my parents' house. I did not realize they were there to meet for the escape room. My sister and her best friend were sitting on the back deck. I had gone into the kitchen to get a drink. When I was heading back to the deck, they were putting the sliding screen door back onto its tracks, as it must have come off. I took one look at the door and it looked different and I became suspicious. I thought they were clones and had swapped the original screen door with a new one that did not lock. This was to make it easier to break into the house. I kept quiet and sat on the chair on the back deck. They were talking about the escape room. And I said, "Oh, you're going to that now? Why didn't you tell me?" My sister hesitated and then with a look of worry and concern replied, "yeah, I'm sorry I didn't know you still wanted to go." At that point I was upset and didn't want to go anymore, especially not with clones. Obviously looking back now I understand that my family was not trying to exclude me but that they knew I was in no mental capacity to go at the time, as something like that would have exacerbated my already severe paranoia.

One thing my dad often did at night was listen to music on the computer. One night he was sitting on the couch in the living room with his music. I noticed a gigantic bug, at least two inches long, on the ceiling behind him. I believed that the bug was watching what he was doing. And feeding information to the bad guys. I was afraid to say anything about the bug. I would just pace back and forth - keeping my eye on it. I often thought that the songs he listened to were songs that he actually wrote and sold to the artists singing them. One song in particular he used to play was "Denise" by Randy and the Rainbows. He always told me to listen to it with him. Given my thoughts, I started to think that my dad had actually written the song "Denise" about a secret lover he had in the past that my mom did not know about. Thinking back to my first episode, I thought about the woman in the visiting room at ECMC the one day and started to think that she was my dad's secret lover. I started to connect the two ideas. I thought that Denise was the woman in the visiting room that day and my dad wrote the song "Denise" about her.

When I would smoke on the front porch, I would often look at the stars. Every night I would notice this one particular star in the sky. I began to think that it wasn't really a star and that it was actually a spaceship. I believed that clones were on the spaceship due to its placement in the sky, which was right above our house. I believed they were listening to my family, my thoughts, and were trying to control the environment in which I was living. I would always stare at it when I was on the porch at night. I thought they had a satellite linked to our Amazon Alexa that allowed them to listen to what was going on in the house.

I would often be up in the middle of the night. One of the things I would watch on T.V. was Time Warner Cable News. I started to think that the news station was actually located on the satellite spaceship hovering above our house. I remember specifically one night the news anchor was talking and he got a concerned look on his face and it turned red. I immediately thought that as he was reporting the news story, he was being shown footage of me on one screen and footage of my family being beaten up at ECMC on another screen. I believed the concerned look on his face was due to the fact that I appeared oblivious to what was happening to my family.

Our porch had a green light on it. I noticed one day that our neighbors across the street had put up a green light on their porch. I thought this was a signal for me to know that they were trustworthy. I also noticed Neighborhood Watch signs on a few of the neighbors' lawns. One of them was a neighbor who my dad had talked to recently. Like the green porch light, the signs also gave me the impression that those select neighbors were not clones and that they were safe to talk to if need be.

I remember watching the T.V. game show Jeopardy and thinking that the contestants' achievements translated to the real world. There was always one contestant that I considered to be a good contestant. Depending on their name, what they were wearing, or what they did, would determine who needed to win in my mind. I remember one day, one of the contestants had the same name as my mother. Therefore, I thought she was the one that needed to win to bring positivity to the world. Another time it was the contestant wearing a blue shirt.

There was one thought I had developed in my mind. It was the idea that the left eye was a powerful gateway. I believed that if you looked through someone's left eye, you could delve into their soul. When I finally felt comfortable leaving the house, I went to the bookstore Barnes and Noble, where I happened to stumble upon a puzzle of an owl. Completing puzzles has always been an activity that my mother and I enjoyed doing together. And this puzzle in particular stood out to me for two reasons. The fact that the puzzle was an image of an owl attracted my attention. This related back to my first episode and the significance that the owl and the Goddess

Athena had to me. But not only was the puzzle an owl, I also noticed that the right eye of the owl had a black ring around it, whereas the left eye had a red ring around it. The fact that the owl had a red ring around it's left eye amplified and confirmed my thoughts of the left eye as being special. This puzzle exuded positive vibes to me. I quickly grabbed the puzzle off the shelf and headed home to complete it with my mother. Once we completed it, I left it assembled on the dining room table for weeks to add positive energy inside our house.

This state of mind I was in, this state of near constant delusion and paranoia, continued on for about a week before is started to slowly get better. With time and medication, the intensity did start to decrease, however I did still have random bouts of paranoia here and there. For example, towards the end of my episode, I had an appointment with my counselor and my psychiatrist. I remember when I went to the lobby, which was in one wing of the building, I heard a girl scream from the other wing of the building. I thought people were being tortured in the opposite wing of the building and I was afraid to be there.

I also remember having fear creep in when I was at one of my other visits. The switch to turn the light on in the bathroom was actually a knob that when turned it prompted a timer, allowing the light to stay on for the duration of the timer. The more you turned the knob the longer the light would stay lit in the bathroom. When I went into the bathroom and turned the knob for the light, irrationality kicked in and I thought I had just set the timer for a bomb in the building. I remember repeatedly going back to the bathroom during my visit to turn the knob so the light would not shut off. In my mind, when the light turned off, the bomb in the building would explode.

As you can imagine, being in this constant state of paranoia and delusion had become exhausting. Hopefully reading through these examples of my thoughts during that time was able to give some insight into what it can be like inside the mind of a person with paranoid and irrational thoughts. It can be a dark and scary place, and a difficult place to be pulled out of. And hopefully it also showed that an episode doesn't just end with the snap of a finger and in the blink of an eye. Coming out of psychosis usually happens gradually, and the thoughts, though they may diminish, can still linger for quite some time.

With regular counseling and psychiatrist visits and a higher dose of medication, I was eventually able to overcome the episode I had just experienced. My mind stabilized over time. I continued with recovery and I do so until this day. Recovery in itself has been its own journey. And if anything, it has been the most important part of my journey.

"Pacing from all of these warped thoughts
My heart skips a beat
I have to control these emotions
Gotta get back on my feet"
-b. amber stark

Section IV
RECOVERY: THE GOOD FIGHT

FIRST STRETCH OF RECOVERY

After experiencing three episodes, I've met the recovery frontline a few times. In fact, I think recovery remains a constant battle. My initial recovery following my first episode seemed to be the hardest recovery point out of all three episodes that I had. I imagine it was due to the fact that it was just that - the first time. I had turned down a new avenue in my life's journey. I was not sure how to navigate what I just went through. Not knowing where this experience would lead me in the future. What did this all mean? What would people think of me?

I think my first episode was the most traumatic in terms of affecting my brain. Looking back, I think there were several signs and symptoms that I experienced in the month leading up to my first break. However, the signs tend to be subtle at first. Especially if you do not know what to look for. And also, the irrational thoughts seemed very real to me, so I was not able to differentiate them from rational thoughts. And therefore, not able to realize anything might be wrong. This led me to believe that what I was thinking was real. Also, because the duration of experiencing symptoms lasted for weeks, I think it contributed to the greater degree of trauma to my brain compared to my second and third episodes, which were shorter.

The symptoms are so subtle for a period of time until the onset of a full-blown episode hits you out of nowhere like a tidal wave. I never really was able to notice the subtle signs until I actually experienced them and was looking back on everything. After having the first episode and experiencing irrational thoughts and feelings, it was easier for me to recognize those types of thoughts when they occurred again in the future. Because I was now familiar with how it felt, I was more quickly able to identify when my mind was starting to spiral out of control again. Therefore, I think this led to me identifying the irrational thoughts and treating them sooner for my second and third episodes. The sooner I was able to treat these symptoms, the more I was able to prevent my brain from experiencing longer periods of trauma, resulting in the ability to bounce back quicker.

From experience, I think that mental health ailments seem to fall on a spectrum. Paranoia can be either positive or negative. And can fall anywhere in between. What I mean by negative paranoia is experiencing paranoia that manifests in a way where I felt terrified and would try to physically hide from the fears I was having. For example, cowering in a corner or hiding under a blanket. Paranoia that made me feel like if I "made the wrong move" bad things would happen. Positive paranoia, on the other hand, manifests in a way where the fear still exists, but there is a sense of invincibility where I felt I had the power and ideas to help battle through the fearful thoughts I was having. For me, I feel that I experienced negative paranoia in my first episode and positive paranoia in my second episode, or my manic state. Referring to the mental health ailments on a spectrum, I think there can also be a combination of both types of paranoia in different degrees. To clarify, I think I experienced a mix of both negative and positive paranoia during my third episode. The paranoia I experienced had me terrified where I felt like hiding, but I always tried to remain calm and overcome what I was thinking and feeling.

Anxiety can also be experienced in different ways. And even though anxiety is a common ailment people experience, I do not think anxiety can be pinpointed as one single type of feeling. This concept of feeling is a little harder to put into words. Personally, I experienced anxiety across the board throughout all three episodes and to this day. But it didn't always feel the same. For example, one of the times that I was having an anxiety attack, I had a very uncomfortable feeling in my shoulder blades. So uncomfortable that it was painful. I literally wanted to rip out of my own skin. Other times, I would get jitters in my brain and body, making it hard for me to sit still and relax. So, with anxiety I'd feel a variety of different physical pain or sensations. Regardless of how the anxiety manifested, it was always mentally draining and crippling.

One thing I remember from the first recovery was being highly medicated. Days following my first hospital visit, I felt extremely wiped out and tired. This lasted for months. In the beginning I was sleeping a lot. If I was not sleeping, I felt run down and I had no energy. I would lie on the couch like a vegetable. There was no life in me. I had been prescribed a high dose of Risperidone to help control the psychotic features of my episode (the paranoia, hallucinations, and delusions). I was prescribed Ativan to help control the anxiety that would creep in. I was not a fan of being on these medications, namely the high dose of Risperidone. I was also wary of the Ativan considering it is a benzodiazepine, which is a very addictive drug class.

I had frequent visits with my mental health counselor, my substance abuse counselor, and my psychiatrist following my first episode. Over the course of my meetings with my substance abuse counselor, we discussed the importance of sobriety and the role it plays in maintaining a healthy and stable mind. I remember talking to her about blacking out after drinking alcohol, which is something I often experienced in years past. We discussed the danger and harm of blacking out, and the detriment it can have to a person's mental health. With all of this in mind, in the beginning of my treatment I remained totally clean. And when my substance abuse counselor would ask me at our weekly visits if I had consumed alcohol or smoked pot, I was able to answer with honesty that I hadn't. However, after a few months of treatment I became more lax and started to drink a single beer on occasion. I confessed this to my counselor at our next few visits. She expressed her disappointment each time but also had a discussion with me as to why I may have made the choice. She said that just the simple fact that there was beer in the house possibly triggered a temptation that I gave in to. She also informed me that if I were to keep drinking and not take treatment seriously then I would not be eligible to remain in treatment. Abstaining from substances, in my case alcohol and pot, was a requirement to receive the treatment. It was a No Tolerance program. She reiterated the importance of staying sober and how it would affect my medications and my progress in recovering. I remember the effect that her disappointment, as well as her insight, had on me following my confessions of drinking. I realized that if I was serious about recovering successfully, I had to make a change in lifestyle. I had to quit the alcohol and pot. So, for months following, I did just that. I would get tested and my drug tests would come back clean. I abstained from drinking, eventually to the point where I completed the substance abuse program.

Aside from substance abuse counseling I also received mental health counseling. I discussed things about my personal life like my family, my job, my hobbies (or lack thereof), my social life, and my struggles. We would pinpoint my weaknesses and try to develop ways for me to become stronger. We would discuss strategies and techniques to combat anxiety. One way to deescalate anxiety is to simply engage in deep breathing. Close your eyes, breathe in and out slowly - in through your nose and out through your mouth. Another way is to focus in on what is around you. If you are in a room, or if you're outside, look around and focus in on three things. Pay attention to the details of what you're looking at. For example, with a picture you could focus in on the color, the texture and the story it tells. Give your attention to these details for a few minutes. This will re-direct your mind and distract you from the thoughts that were causing the anxiety in the first place. Another way is to sit straight up in a chair with your feet flat on the ground with good posture. Start at your feet, focusing in on them, the way they are touching the ground. Move up your legs, to your hips, to your arms, neck and head. Focus in on your face and how your eyes are closed. Another example includes focusing in on the chair you're sitting on. Is it soft? Is it hard? Does it rock or recline? Focus in on the sounds around you. Whether it be the sound of a fan close by, a muffled voice in the next room or the sound of traffic passing by. Focusing in on things in your surroundings is a way to alleviate anxiety levels because it gets you out of your own head and forces you to be present. Another method my counselor told me about is to take an hour-glass timer and flip it upside down. Pay attention to the sand falling through, collecting into a mound at the bottom. Focus on how the pile grows bigger on the bottom and gets smaller at the top. The mound looks like a mountain. Where the sand is falling through, it starts to create a recessed imprint where a hole is beginning to form. Paying attention to the minute details of everything happening within the hour-glass occupies the mind and controls your anxiety. These are all techniques that can help calm you. Engaging in them can help put you back in control of your mind. Other techniques I've used to help combat my anxiety include listening to music or singing a song, coloring, and doing exercises such as crunches, push-ups, handstands and yoga poses.

Aside from my counselors, I had a psychiatrist that I met with monthly who helped manage my medications. We would have brief meetings to follow up on how things were going and how I was feeling, as well as to renew scripts if my medications were running low. Now, before I went into the hospital for the first time, I had been taking Lexapro, which is an antidepressant. This medication was initially prescribed to me by my primary physician based on a depressed mental state I had experienced, which most likely stemmed from the loss of my great aunt and my childhood dog. When I was admitted into the hospital, I was taken off the Lexapro and prescribed the Risperidone and Ativan. Once I was discharged from the hospital, I continued to take the Risperidone and Ativan. I remember at my initial meeting with my psychiatrist I told him that I didn't like how the Ativan made me feel. It would help battle my anxiety but when it wore off, I would experience greater degrees of anxiety. He agreed to stop the Ativan. Aside from the anxiety, I was also experiencing akathisia. Akathisia, or pacing, is a side effect experienced from taking a high dose of Risperidone. So, to offset the akathisia, I was prescribed the medication Cogentin. I continued with the combination of Risperidone and Cogentin. However, I still continued to experience a lot of anxiety, which led to an outlet I would later regret. I picked up the bad habit of smoking cigarettes. Up until that point in my life, I had never smoked before. But unfortunately, it would help calm my nerves when my anxiety would escalate. Again, it is something I deeply regret and it is important to remember that there are other healthier modes to help battle anxiety than picking up the unhealthy habit of smoking cigarettes.

Now I am the type of person that rarely takes medication, not even an aspirin in the case of a headache. I was just never comfortable with the notion of being dependent on an external substance to heal or aid my body. So, the fact that I had to be on certain medications at all really bothered me. Aside from already not being a fan of medications in general, the way these new medications were making me feel was an issue for me. I remember going into an appointment one time, about two months into treatment, and explaining how I did not like how I felt on the medication. I felt so flat and like a nobody. Now, instead of feeling too much, like I did with the paranoia, fear, and delusions - I started to not feel anything. That is with the exception of crippling anxiety. I was a vegetable. I felt no emotions. I felt as if my mind was paralyzed. Paralyzed. Nothing came in and nothing went out. And I felt this way for months. And I hated it. It was hard to be around other people other than my immediate family because I just couldn't interact and didn't interact. I felt as if others would think of me as being weird. I was on such a high dose of Risperidone that I would sleep all the time. When I was awake, it wouldn't matter because it was like I wasn't even there. Absolutely no interactions. I was just there - I merely existed. There were things I could do to help my mental state, such as exercise, but there was no life in me or energy to do it. It was not really an option.

When I mentioned my concerns about being on the high dose of medication, my psychiatrist said he understood my frustrations. But he explained to me that my brain is very fragile and had undergone severe trauma from the episode I had experienced and needed at least six months to begin healing and to recover properly. So, I would have to stay on the higher dose of Risperidone for about another four months. Being on the high dose of Risperidone would help prevent any more trauma to my brain and prevent another episode from occurring. It would give my brain the time it needed to heal. At the time it was mid-March. So, he said about mid-June I could consider weaning down the Risperidone. I listened to what he said and trusted that it was the best path. I continued with my treatment in all three areas (substance abuse counseling, mental health counseling, and seeing the psychiatrist) for the months to follow, working hard to tackle my issues. I was diligent about what I should do, what I should not do, and focused on really trying hard. Because it was not easy. I had good days, and I had really bad days. But I kept pushing and I listened to the professionals I was seeing - and most importantly I did my part. They can only listen to your story and guide you. But it's up to you to carry yourself and make the changes necessary to pull all the way through. Being an advocate for yourself and being honest about how you're feeling, along with perseverance, having a positive mindset and knowing that things can get better are all keys to a successful treatment

I continued with my recovery - attending counseling, meeting with my psychiatrist and taking my medications. Further into recovery I again spoke to my psychiatrist about not being a fan of the medication and not liking the way it was making me feel. I could not take the flat feeling, the feeling of being a nobody. Not to mention I had gained 34 pounds from being on the medication in just a few months' time, which added to me feeling depressed. But he again reminded me of the medicine's importance to my brain's recovery and I continued to stay the course.

After months of meetings with my psychiatrist, working with my counselors and maintaining a healthy work habit, it was decided that I was making progress mentally. I had also stayed clean from drinking and smoking pot. I met the expectations of staying clean for six months and I was finally able to conclude treatment with my chemical dependency counselor on May 20, 2014. In June of 2014, my psychiatrist finally decided it was okay to lower my medication. This is a process that needs to be done carefully and gradually over months to help prevent adverse side effects and cause minimal withdrawal. Therefore, the Risperidone was lowered by .5 mg to begin the weaning process and the Cogentin was switched to a PRN, or a "take as needed" basis. After being on the lower dose for a month or so, I found that I was feeling a little more alive. I slowly gained interest in things again and would interact with others. I wasn't feeling as flat as I was when I initially started my recovery.

One negative thing I experienced that I thought was a result from lowering the Risperidone was that I would randomly get "brain zaps" in the weeks initially following. The best way I can explain the zaps would be comparable to the sensation you get from an electrical shock, and they would happen randomly and suddenly. This was just something I learned to tolerate. On a more positive note, lowering the dose enabled me to eliminate the Cogentin because I no longer experienced akathisia on the lower dose of Risperidone. Also, my anxiety was not as high or frequent as it had been.

By the end of August 2014, I seemed to be maintaining stability and doing well. Time between my appointments grew longer which was an indicator that things were going well. At this point, I began to meet with my mental health counselor once every 4-6 weeks. And I would meet with my psychiatrist even more sporadically, mainly for medication management and brief check-ups to make sure all was well as I continued the process of titrating off the Risperidone. At counseling, I would continue to gain more strategies, techniques, and tools to help improve my mental health and continue to fight my "demons," like anxiety and depressed thoughts. My counselor suggested watching TED talks. One talk in particular that she thought I would like was called "Cloudy with a Chance of Joy" by Gavin

Pretor-Pinney. In the talk the speaker mentions how we always associate clouds with negativity. We apply the idea of clouds with a "doom and gloom metaphor." We see them as getting in the way of the Sun. So, it is easy to compare them with obstructions in life. But he goes on to mention that if we sit back and appreciate the clouds and their beauty, we may see that the clouds blocking the Sun can form a beautiful figure. It could be said that I considered my first episode as being a "cloud" in my life. After applying the information from the talk, it made me realize that maybe my episode was a blessing in disguise. And that I should learn to focus on the silver linings when things seem "cloudy" and find the beauty even in the worst of situations. This led me to think about having a positive attitude no matter what life throws my way. Another thing I took away from the talk was to take the time to appreciate the beauty around you without getting caught up in the "busy" stuff. This talk mentioned not getting caught up in the "what I should have done" and "what I gotta do," and to just live in the present. I think this helped me with my anxiety. I also feel that taking the time to appreciate what's around you and to find the beauty in what's in front of you helps alleviate anxiety and depression and adds to a happier self.

By December of 2014, I was down to taking 1 mg of Risperidone a day. I felt feelings and emotions again. Some days were good and some days were bad. My mood would fluctuate from feeling down for a couple of days followed by a couple of days of feeling happy. No longer paralyzed. I was just happy to feel feelings. I found myself interacting with people. Conversations and engaging with others had started to become easier. Things with work were going well. I felt human again.

Aside from feeling better as far as a stable mind goes, there were other things I wanted to improve on. One thing I wanted to combat was the lingering addiction to cigarettes I had developed. At the time I started, I did not see it as an issue because as mentioned before, it helped me get through spells of anxiety. But as time went on, a smoker was not who I wanted to be. I also remained self-conscious because of the weight I had put on due to the medication. But I would tell myself that it was only temporary and that it could be changed.

January of 2015 arrived. I started out the new year by going to the gym frequently. A resolution I made for myself. Around the second week in January, I started having some health issues - one of them being the excessive need to use the bathroom. So excessive that I ended up losing almost 10 pounds in less than two weeks. A catch-22, as I was happy about the weight loss but suspicious of the frequent bathroom trips and rapid weight loss. While doing some research to try to figure out what the cause could have been, I stumbled upon the fact that my Risperidone was being supplied by a different manufacturer than before. I had suspicions that the different manufacturer was the cause behind the frequent bathroom breaks. About a week after taking the new refill of the Risperidone, I had started to have these issues. I started to think that the medication from the new manufacturer had given me parasites. From that point, I decided I no longer wanted to take the medication which I discussed with my psychiatrist. Therefore, he gave me a schedule of how to completely taper off of it. But even after being off the medication, I continued to lose weight. I went from weighing 155 pounds in December, to 130 pounds by the end of January, to eventually reaching 105 pounds by May. I experienced random bruising all over my legs. I had stomach issues. I would get chest pain frequently. My anxiety was increasing, which I was no longer treating with the Ativan. There were a number of issues that I experienced. I researched the symptoms online, which was a bad idea and led me to believe the worst-case scenarios as to why I was experiencing these issues. And looking back I believe that some of the issues were linked to the anxiety I was experiencing. Aside from these health issues though, I felt that I was otherwise in a good place mentally and mood-wise, as I was now pretty much medication-free, feeling more alert, and had lost a significant amount of weight. I felt comfortable enough with my progress to the point where I unfortunately started falling back into old habits. My progress had lulled me into an almost false sense of security, and by April of 2015 I had reached another low point as far as decision-making. I had regressed back to smoking pot and drinking on a weekly basis. I started smoking pot again to self-medicate since I was no longer taking Ativan for the anxiety. Eventually, I slipped back into a hole of self-medicating and being ultra-dependent on the pot. It started out that I was using the pot to dampen the anxiety. But in turn I think it led to more anxiety. It was a sick cycle of suffering from anxiety, then using the pot to mask it, to then just come down and suffer more anxiety.

But again, even in dealing with those issues, I still felt good. Definitely better than I had in the months prior. I didn't see the anxiety as being an issue because I was always masking it, and I was feeling more energized and on top of the world. I didn't realize it at the time but looking back I think I was suffering from a hypomanic state. I was just super happy and I was making associations left and right. Everything I thought about related to something else and had really deep meaning for me. And as I covered earlier, my hypomanic state eventually spiraled into a full-blown manic episode in July of 2015, effectively ending my first period of recovery. My family described this time to me as particularly hard because it was difficult for them to watch me go from doing so well, from having made so much progress and finally getting back to my old self, to then essentially losing all that progress. As if my recovery was almost like me climbing a mountain, steadily climbing towards that peak, making such great improvements and progress, only to get to the top and abruptly fall from the cliff again.

"It's not about the ups and downs but more the highs and lows
   A stable mind with a peaceful soul and pinpointing the perfect dose
   Easing a warped and twisted mind
   And stabilizing the feelings that are intertwined
   Tweaking all the highs and lows at the onset of the very first sign"
-b. amber stark

SECOND STRETCH OF RECOVERY

My second stretch of recovery began after my two-week stay at BryLin following my second episode. This time around I was again prescribed Risperidone and Ativan with the addition of Lithium. Lithium is a mood stabilizer and was added to my prescriptions to help manage the mania I experienced in my second episode. This included my elated mood, invincible sense of self, lack of sleep and feelings of grandeur. I believe that since my energy level was so high due to the mania, the Risperidone did not have the same dampening effect as it did for the first stretch of recovery. The Ativan, again, was used to treat my anxiety.

One tool I used following my second hospital stay was recording my thoughts to paper. I would carry a notepad and pen around with me. Everything I wrote down was dated, along with the time of day. Kind of like verses in the Bible. I wrote mostly song lyrics from songs that I listened to throughout the day. I would record thoughts that the songs would trigger. Each time-stamped song lyric or thought was usually brief. I used music a lot to help me get through my days. I would grab a hold of a lyric from a song and carry it away in my hypomanic mind. I would often think that certain songs were about specific people in my life. That certain songs were written specifically for my life. Aside from self-help from music, writing, coloring, and walks, I began the treatment program called OnTrack. As, mentioned before, this was a program where I had the option to meet with a counselor at my home if needed. It also offered a hotline to call in a crisis for immediate attention to whatever the issue may be. Through the program, I was linked with a counselor and a psychiatrist. Immediately following my hospital stay I would meet with my counselor weekly. After a few weeks of treatment, I was also linked to a women's group for offsite therapy sessions at an alternate location.

I remember one thing I discussed with my counselor was the importance of honesty. Particularly, the importance of me being honest with my counselor and psychiatrist in order to receive appropriate and effective treatment. During one of my group sessions, mid-September 2015, we were given the task of writing a brief essay to share in group. Therefore, I decided to focus on the topic of the importance of honesty. I presented the following essay, which was written in a hypomanic state, in group the following week.

"Honesty with Self, Honesty with Others"

"I lived to learn that honesty is the best policy. Growing up I often heard this and was taught this time and time again. However, I had to learn the hard way. Why bother trying to live a lie when all it really does is complicate things. Nowadays, I like to keep things simple- being honest. That's simple. Some may beg to differ but in reality when you lie it's hard to keep track of your story. Stick to the truth and your story never changes. If you find it hard to be honest, maybe it's a way of showing something within you may need some work. But realizing that is the first step in improving yourself - whether it's a lie to yourself or others. I think we can all agree that lies just contribute to disrespecting yourself and/or others. I have lied in the past but it's not something I do anymore. I've learned that things are a lot smoother and way simpler when the truth is told. Lies create problems and force people to build walls that prevent them from getting hurt. Lies ruin relationships. Lies also feed others negative ideas about your character. I think it all comes down *to one mantra: the Golden Rule - treat others the way you would like to be treated. Before lying ask yourself how you would feel if you were on the other side of that lie. Chances are you would find negative connotations. Why take the chance of breaking a good relationship with another because of a petty lie? Respect and conversations are key. The key to someone else's heart and soul is honesty. Lying is a lost key that gets you nowhere but into trouble. Another side of honesty is of course with one's self. In my current situation, it is up to me to be honest with my counselors and psychiatrist in order to receive the appropriate help and assistance I need. Lying is negative and just snowballs into a toxic snowman. One lie leads to other lies, and before you know it, you get stressed trying to keep up with your lies. Keep your story and life simple by being honest. Honesty builds character and a jolly happy soul. So, it's your choice to either build an abominable snowman or Frosty the Snowman. Who would you rather "chill" out with?"*

Coming to terms with how I was feeling and being able to express it to my counselor and psychiatrist was extremely important. Writing was a way to help me do this. At the end of August of 2015 I decided to write about my mental health experiences from the past couple of years. So, at that point I started to journal about my first episode, which would eventually become part of this book. I used writing as a tool to help me come to terms with what was going on with me. My psychiatrist had told me that I was being treated for Bipolar Disorder. So many negative things came over me when I heard this classification. Especially the thought of what other people were going to think of me. I constantly thought to myself that it wasn't true. I didn't seem to fit the description of what I thought bipolar meant. I imagined a person who had severe mood swings. Someone who would be happy one second, and the next second be angry and lashing out at others. That wasn't really a good descriptor for what I had been experiencing. I did some research online. I watched documentaries on people who suffered from Bipolar. I just could not come to terms with it. I couldn't relate to what they described feeling. In particular, the lows of the mental disorder. I did have bad days where I felt depressed, even to the point of having suicidal thoughts. But not to the degree that the individuals in these videos were describing. I had experienced mania, paranoia, delusions and anxiety. I started to think that I was being prescribed for the wrong thing, if I even needed medication at all. I did find a description online of Bipolar presenting symptoms of paranoia and delusions and a manic state. Dr. Tracey Marks stated, "Mania is a defining characteristic of Bipolar Disorder." After I stumbled upon that information, along with my psychiatrist explaining to me how it's the best classification for what I had experienced, I began to come to terms with the fact that maybe this really was how to describe my mental health.

It's important to note that my psychiatrist told me not to get caught up in the diagnosis. Mental health is difficult in the sense that mental health classifications can share common ground and overlapping symptoms, which can make it hard to pinpoint an exact disorder. For example, it can be hard to differentiate between Bipolar Disorder with psychotic features and Schizoaffective Disorder because of their similarities. The most important part when dealing with mental health issues is getting proper treatment that works and allows one to lead a fulfilling life.

Treatment carried on. My mind was stabilizing. I was dedicated to abstaining from drinking. And pot was not even a thought in my mind. Unfortunately, cigarettes were still a thing for me. Similar to the first recovery, I was constantly trying to work at lowering my medications. As my sessions with my psychiatrist and counselor were going well, my psychiatrist said it was alright for me to taper down my medication. So, I took a small step down. My sister got engaged in December and we had an engagement party planned for her in January. I had a conversation with my psychiatrist about being able to consume alcohol at the party. He said he didn't recommend it and said that having a drink or two would be fine for special occasions ONLY. So, at the engagement party I did have a single beer. It was my first beer since June. But even after being told I could have a couple of drinks for special occasions, I still didn't care to take the chance. I was pretty focused on maintaining a stable mind, especially because another one of my sisters was due to have a baby in June of 2016. So, I rarely would consume alcohol, if at all. Things had been going well and I was able to taper down my Risperidone again as well as the Lithium. After tapering down I lost a lot of weight again. I went from weighing 135 pounds in December to 105 pounds by the time June 2016 came around. June arrived and it was a month of mixed emotions. It marked one year since my boyfriend of ten years had walked out, which was a downer. But it was also the birth of my first niece. I was thrilled to be a first-time aunt. So, I continued on with my recovery with everything seeming to go well. I still battled typical emotions of everyday life, but nothing seemed to be extreme. No mania or depression which was good.

The end of June 2016 arrived and I was feeling good and confident in my recovery. It had been about a year since my second episode and I still hadn't been drinking. I had made plans to go out with my friend, Rhee. I remember suffering from a horrible headache early on in the night before heading to the bar, to the point that I had to lie down on her couch. A side note, I didn't know it at the time, but since then I've started to link that specific type of headache I had that night as a precursor to an episode. I didn't want to disappoint Rhee, so I fought through the pain and went out to the bar. This was the point where, as mentioned earlier in the book, I met the young man at the bar and began to grow paranoid and freaked out by our conversation. The days following would be the start to my third episode and yet another end to a period of recovery.

It is important to note that throughout my whole second stretch of recovery I did not drink alcohol or smoke pot. I had learned my lesson from my first recovery and didn't want to take the chance. But even with abstaining from drugs and alcohol, I still slipped into a third episode. This was proof to my family and me that it wasn't just the external factors of drugs and alcohol that had contributed to my prior episodes, and that it was indeed internal brain chemistry, and likely genetics, that was a prominent factor to my mental health issues.

When I slipped into my third episode, it brought up a lot of questions for my family and me. And some scary possibilities. It couldn't be ignored that things seemed to be happening in a sort of pattern now. Almost like a repeating cycle. The time between each episode seemed to be just about exactly a year. We began to wonder if this would just be an annual thing. A cycle. That maybe I would have an episode every single summer. And that was a scary and debilitating thought. And it made going into my third stretch of recovery that much more loaded with meaning and purpose. I was more determined than ever to get well - and more importantly, to stay well. I knew it would be a challenge, and probably the fight of my life. But I was ready to do it all again. To once again tackle recovery and to fight the good fight, for a third time.

"I'll stop you from creeping in my shadow
   Free myself from the stress you like to hold hands with
   Shield you with my strength, my bare feet on the gravel
   Prevent you from stealing me from my next breath"
-b. amber stark

THIRD STRETCH OF RECOVERY

Throughout the span of my three episodes, it was like I was on a merry-go-round of increasing and decreasing medication. I'd be able to slowly wean down, but once I started regressing, I would once again have to increase the medication. So, immediately following the third episode, I was back to a higher dose of Risperidone. I felt a little flat again, but I knew it was what was necessary. With the first episode, it was harder to have to take medication because I did not realize how helpful it could be. But by the third episode I knew it was what was necessary to get myself back to the other side, back to a stable mind. And I knew it was only temporary. I maintained the higher dose for a number of weeks. I started to put weight back on again slowly. Things remained stable for months and again conversation of lowering the dose came to the table. I decided to take things a little slower this time around. I decided to lower the dose, but not to rush the process. This time around I was more focused on doing what was right for my mental health and not getting caught up in the idea that I did not want to be on medication. My experience taught me the importance of being patient even when you feel frustrated with the process of trying to wean off medication. I remained on the same dose through Fall, Winter, and Spring, with everything going well. Well enough that lowering my dose again was a possibility. But my sister's wedding was around the corner, and I did not want to cause any issues as far as experiencing an episode. So, I told my psychiatrist that I did not want to taper down again until after the wedding. Not to mention, summer time seemed to be when I was more likely to experience an episode, judging by past cycles. So, I wanted to be extra cautious to avoid any issues. Therefore, I continued with my medications at the dose I was at to be safe.

The wedding passed and the summer passed without incident. All was well. Making it through the Summer of 2017 without any issues was an important milestone for me because it would mark the first time I had gone more than a year without experiencing an episode. It spoke volumes to me in terms of recovery. As well as quality of life. Not that I was totally out of the woods, but I was in a good place. I spent time slowly continuing to journal, documenting my experiences. I had two goals. One was to try to quit smoking for the fourth time, and the other was to lower my medication when I was ready. So that Fall, November 25, 2017, would mark the last day I smoked a cigarette. I was committed to quitting for a number of reasons. One being that my second niece was due to be born following the New Year and I wanted to be smoke-free by then. So, I fought the battle and I conquered the addiction for the most part. I say for the most part because once in a while the urge does still creep in. But, as time has passed, it is now definitely easier to say no than it was in the beginning of the fight. And as far as lowering my medication, that came a little later as I did not want to make too many changes at once. By May 2018, I met my second goal of lowering my medication and I still hadn't had a cigarette since November of 2017. At that point, along with journaling, I began writing poems. Poems on topics including mental health, love, heartbreak, nature, life's choices, and other musings. I seemed to be in a really good place and I did not want to interrupt that. I remained on the same dose of my medication from Spring of 2018 to December of 2020.

There were only a couple of instances in between that time where I experienced a bout of paranoia here and there, but that would only last about a day. When these bouts of paranoia would happen, I would simply increase the dose of Risperidone for a couple of days if I could not control it before lowering it again, as advised by my psychiatrist. I've been able to identify early symptoms and manage them which prevents me from suffering from a full-blown episode. So far, anyway.

I think it is important to note that my first hospital stay lasted three weeks, my second hospital stay lasted about two weeks, and I came out of my third episode in about ten days. So, every time I experienced an episode, the duration shortened each time. I saw that as an improvement in the sense that my brain was able to heal more quickly each time. And I believe there was one major reason for the quicker recovery. Knowing what to look for and being able to recognize and verbalize the symptoms I was having sooner, allowed me to be proactive and increase my medicine dosage before too much trauma was done to my brain. This goes to show how being able to identify triggers and signs is vitally important in terms of recovery and maintaining stability. I was able to communicate the issues I was having which allowed for immediate treatment. I remember bouncing back quicker the third time compared to the first two times.

Some early indications of a potential episode for me include experiencing odd smells and/or a specific type of severe headache. Some early signs I try to tackle include extreme anxiety, lack of or little need for sleep, and suspicious thoughts. If I have anxiety I can't manage on my own, I will take Ativan if necessary. But I will never take Ativan for more than three days in a row. This is to avoid becoming dependent on it. If I find that I am experiencing little need for sleep I will try to tweak my schedule and lie down earlier to help me fall asleep. I'll use weekends to really try and manipulate my sleep schedule and keep it on track. I am getting at least six hours of sleep a night. Suspicious thoughts are basically paranoia, but to a lesser degree. So, I try not to feed into the suspicion, and instead talk through it with someone I trust in order to prevent it from snowballing to severe paranoia. It reminds me of the movie *A Beautiful Mind*, where at the end of the movie the character discusses his demons as basically always being present in his life, but he chooses not to pay attention to them. That's how paranoia is for me. Sometimes it's there, I just try not to feed into the thoughts when they creep in. It is like I had to train myself to ward off the paranoid thoughts. I think by doing this I control my thoughts. I think it is important to learn to control the thoughts because if you don't, they will eventually control you. Now, if it gets to a point where I can't control it, I immediately talk to my family about it. They tell me whether my thoughts are rational or not. But overall, I'm in control the majority of the time. Which is an important step to surpass in recovery. Even though I know recovery will always remain a battle.

"Living with a tight mind
No room for breathing
Memories on the rewind
Thoughts that are deceiving

Speeding on this mental highway
Stuck in overdrive
Drowning in insanity
Fighting to survive

My family gives support
That gets me through the day
As I search for the mind control
To make everything okay

Grateful for their presence
In taking care of me
Providing strength and courage
As I pray on bended knee"
-b. amber stark

Section V
LIFEBUOYS

While most of this book is comprised of my personal journey and experiences, I think it's also important to discuss the effect that a mental health episode can have on the loved ones of an individual suffering. To recognize how much strength it takes for them to remain standing on their own feet while also supporting and caring for someone who is struggling with mental health issues. I know firsthand how much weight it can be on their shoulders to worry and care, and to want to make everything better. I named this section LIFEBUOYS after the life saving devices because that is what my family has been to me. Throughout my experiences, whenever I've felt I was drowning, when the violent waves of my mental struggles have threatened to crash over me and pull me under, my family is what has kept me afloat. In short, they've saved me many times along this journey. And again, I feel it's important to acknowledge that a mental health episode does not only affect the individual suffering from one. It also affects any friends and family members who are trying to provide support to that person. So, I asked my family to share any insights on their experiences during my episodes. My sister, Ava, wrote a cumulative account of my family's experiences during that time and I've included it below.

I'll never forget that very first night, when B's initial mental health episode first started. And those first few moments when we realized something was really, really wrong. They were some of the scariest and most confusing moments of my life. She had driven to my parent's house in a panic and was suddenly saying very irrational things - things like her boyfriend and roommate were after her, that our family was in danger, that people were following her. She was crying and clearly legitimately terrified. But we couldn't understand what had set this off. We could obviously see that there was no real threat or danger, but when we tried to explain that to her, she wouldn't believe us. She would get quiet for a while, and it was clear that the wheels were turning in her head and she looked very tense and paranoid. She was making veiled and cryptic statements that weren't making any sense. At one point she looked at my sister very suspiciously and asked her why she had gotten the same haircut as her. It almost seemed to be an accusation. It was a peculiar comment that I might've laughed at in any other situation. But at that moment and the way it was stated, it was clear that irrational thoughts and connections had taken hold and that at that point she may not even trust us, her family. It made a cold fear creep into me because it was becoming more and more apparent that her mind had gone completely out of control. As we were all gathered at my parents' house to try to figure out what to do, we felt helpless. It was heartbreaking to see how scared and confused she was, and nothing we said seemed to be able to calm her. It was like no logical thought was really getting through to her. She had a separate reality playing out in her head, and nothing we said could penetrate it or convince her that it wasn't real.

At that point it was like a balancing act for us. We tried our best to present a calm demeanor to her in order to keep her calm. But behind the scenes we were growing increasingly tense and concerned, whispering to each other in panic and trying to figure out what the hell was going on with her. And what we should do about it. This was something we had never experienced before and it was outside our scope of understanding. We really had no prior experience with any sort of mental health issue so we couldn't even recognize that that's what might be going on with her. All we knew is that we were scared and confused and wanted to get her help. We decided that the best course of action was to take her to the hospital, even though we weren't quite sure what we were even taking her there to be treated for. We just knew that when something is wrong with a loved one, that's where you go. Once we got her there and she was evaluated, one of the doctors came out to talk to us. And he put it quite plainly to us. "Yes. She's very sick." Sick. For some reason that word immediately put a pit in my stomach. I had classified in my mind that what she was experiencing was maybe some sort of temporary confusion. Maybe brought on by some sort of exhaustion. Naively, I had thought it was maybe something that would clear up in a couple of hours once she had some time to rest and could clear her head a bit. But it soon became evident that that wouldn't be the case. That this was probably going to be a much longer road. She was sick and would need treatment to get better.

This threw us into the journey that we still continue on today. That day we were suddenly thrown into a world of mental health wards, of different medications, of new terms and codes, and so many other things that were unfamiliar to us. Those first few days were frustrating because it seemed like we were met with a roster of rotating doctors and nurses where it was often difficult to pin down any one doctor and be able to talk to anyone on a consistent basis. Since we had arrived and spoken to that first doctor, no one had really sat down and explained anything to us. We understood B was sick and had to be admitted to the hospital, but we still weren't clear on much else. No one had specifically explained anything as far as a possible diagnosis, prognosis or plan of action. We were just told to be patient and "give the medicine a chance to work." Looking back and having learned a lot since then about mental health and how its diagnosed, I understand more now about why this was probably the case. We now know it's a delicate process where they have to consider things like brain chemistry, and B's personal history in order to determine a baseline and a best course of treatment. We didn't realize that when it comes to mental health, it can take years to reach a formal diagnosis. The reason we probably weren't getting immediate answers was probably because there simply weren't any to give. I'm sure that behind the scenes the doctors were asking B questions and trying to get a grasp of what state her mind and brain might be in. What medication might help to correct whatever was going on in the short-term until they could determine a more concrete diagnosis. But in large part, none of that was really being communicated to us at the time. We still felt mostly in the dark, and were still watching confused and helpless and scared as our loved one's state of mind seemed to be deteriorating. We realized our best option was probably to begin researching and trying to navigate things on our own as well in the meantime. And we were also fortunate because one of B's friends from college was in his residency at that hospital and he became a great resource for us to go to with questions. He did his best to walk us through what was happening with the knowledge that he had of B's situation, and for that we were so grateful.

I remember when it became clear that B would need to stay at the hospital, we requested a formal sit-down with the doctors at ECMC. To try to finally get some solid clarification and guidance on what was going on. Even a name for it. A diagnosis. A plan of action. Anything. Unfortunately, as we would come to learn and as I mentioned before, when it comes to mental illness, those things are not that simple to answer, or at least take a long time to answer. But I do know at one point one of the doctors did use the term "first break." He said that's what B was experiencing - a "first break." So, afterward we went home and we started googling. And started the process of researching. Could this be true? Could this be what was going on - a psychotic break? And the probability that there was an underlying mental illness that was causing it? We thought no, surely we would've noticed something before this, at some point in her life. We would've had an inkling before now if it was something that serious. But once we did some research, there it was. It checked out. "Psychosis is characterized as disruptions to a person's thoughts and perceptions that make it difficult for them to recognize what is real and what isn't." Check. "Three out of 100 people will experience psychosis at some time in their lives." Check. "Psychosis refers to a collection of symptoms that affect the mind, where there has been some loss of contact with reality" Check. "Psychosis often begins in young adulthood when a person is in their late teens to mid-20s." Check. "Psychosis symptoms can be a part of a physical or mental illness that emerge later in life. Other possible causes of psychosis include sleep deprivation, certain prescription medications, and the misuse of alcohol and drugs." The pieces of the puzzle started coming together and the more we looked into it and researched down this path of mental illnesses and disorders of the mind, the more it all fit and made sense. Again, it would be a while before we were actually able to get a solid diagnosis and a name for what was going on, but that was when I think we began to accept that yes, she was sick. She was mentally ill.

It's amazing to me the amount of detail that B is able to recall from her experiences and her time at the hospital. To me that time is more a blur of moments, and I can more clearly and acutely just recall our feelings during that time. Scared. Confused. Exhausted. We felt anguish. Desperation. But I will say there are certain memories that do stick out to me vividly. One of them was during that meeting we requested early on with the doctors at ECMC. When one of the doctors looked at my mom from across the conference room table, with sympathy and compassion. He said he understood how hard it must be to watch your child go through this. To see your child, who up until now had been happy and healthy her whole life, mentally deteriorate before your eyes and being helpless to do much. I just remember my mom burying her face in her hands and the anguish in her voice as she let out a cry. I think the gravity of the situation sank in for her in that moment. I think she was scared for B and what she would have to face going forward. My heart broke for her and I couldn't imagine the feeling of helplessness she must've felt to see her child going through this.

Another moment I recall vividly was during B's hospital stay at ECMC. It was the blanket incident that she described earlier in the book. It had been a few days since we'd brought her to ECMC and her behavior did seem to be getting more and more bizarre. But up until that point it was just mostly strange things that she was saying, and we were learning to get used to it for the time being. We were there that day waiting for her in the common room during visiting hours. Waiting for her to come down and sit and visit with us. She was taking a while to come down from her room and finally when she did, it was one of the more jarring sights I've ever seen. She shuffled into the room very slowly, moving towards us one slow step at a time, with her arms out in front of her slightly and a blanket covering her from head to toe. Like some sort of ghost shuffling slowly towards us. The sight made my hair stand on end and made my stomach drop. It was just such a jarring and bizarre sight to us. It was alarming to see our loved one who for her entire life had been a happy, healthy normal person, to be behaving in this unexplained way. And to not know if she'd come out of it. It was scary. I remember the look on my dad's face. I had never seen it before, but he looked at the nurse with this look of terror and desperation in his eyes. As if he was pleading to her with his eyes - "please help my daughter." During most of that visit B was too scared to come out from underneath the blanket. She just curled up in a ball on the chair next to us, shivering, and refusing to come out. Clearly so terrified. We tried to rub her back and talk to her gently and let her know everything was okay and that she could come out. But she still refused, and pulled the blanket tighter around her frail body. I remember looking at her and watching my family huddled around her helplessly, trying to comfort her, while all looking exhausted and hopelessly worried themselves. And my heart just shattered in that moment. I had to jump up quickly and run to the hallway as tears overwhelmed me. I broke down in the hallway, where one of the nurses comforted me. I just couldn't understand how this all happened so quickly and how our family had gotten to this place seemingly overnight, to a place that I'd never imagined we'd be. And again, my heart just broke for my sister. This was probably one of the worst days we had had up to that point and it really just reiterated how sick she really was. It was a period of uncertainty. It's easier now that things have calmed down and turned out alright, to kind of look back on that time with a more optimistic view. But at the time, things were very uncertain. We didn't know if B would ever come out of the state of mind she was in. We didn't know if the old B would ever return.

I remember going home that night and I broke down to my husband, telling him I was terrified that the old B would never come back. That she was gone beyond return, and this new version of her was permanent. My family was scared and had no idea what to expect going forward or what would happen to B. How long it would take her to come out of this and recover, or if she ever even would at all. At that moment it felt like a death, like the person I'd known and grown up with all my life might not come back. It was a terrifying and devastating feeling.

Another thing I remember from that time is just the feeling of powerlessness and guilt that one of us couldn't stay with her at the hospital. We were only allowed there during visiting hours, and I know it was hard for all of us to have to leave B whenever visiting hours were over. Especially because a mental health hospital can be a scary place to leave a loved one if you're not familiar with one. And if you're not familiar with mental illness in general. Just to see the different behaviors of the patients who may be acting strangely or alarmingly. Looking around that first day, we saw a man with a large cut slashed across his throat stapled together, countless patients shuffling around pacing, yelling and making strange noises, some being restrained or being coaxed to take their medicine. It was overwhelming. And now all of a sudden, our loved one was thrown into the mix among them, behaving in a similar manner. I think we all felt a sense of guilt having to leave her there and having to let go and trust the doctors and to allow the medicine to begin working. Looking back, I do understand it was probably for the best, and it probably did allow each of us to get rest that we too would need but it was still very hard to leave her up there by herself. Obviously now I have a better understanding of mental health, and therefore the fear and stigma I first held for mental health patients and mental health hospitals has been replaced with empathy and understanding. I realize that they are just people who are sick and need help to get better. Just like any other hospital.

Aside from how hard things were that we were experiencing on the inside of the hospital, having to face the outside world during that time was also really difficult. We were all obviously going through hell with this, but we still had to go into work and interact with others and pretty much try to function as normal. And also try to answer questions from others as to what was going on with B. It was hard because it was a delicate topic to really open up to anyone about. Number one because there is not a great amount of understanding among the general population when it comes to mental illness. Things do seem to be improving in that area and trending towards more awareness and less judgement. But there is still a long way to go. And back then, almost ten years ago now, things were even less evolved. So again, it was hard to explain to others exactly what was going on with B. Usually when a loved one suddenly gets diagnosed with a life-changing illness, a physical illness like cancer or leukemia, you usually will tell people and be able to explain why you're going through a hard time. But with a mental illness, it's different. There is a stigma attached, and for some reason a lot of time there's shame attached to it too. So, there was a sense of secrecy and shame involved in all of it as well. When friends or relatives would hear that B was in the hospital and would reach out to us to see if she was okay and what was going on, it was sometimes difficult to answer their questions. For one, because we ourselves were in large part still confused and didn't have answers. And also, for B's sake, we weren't sure we wanted to say too much. We didn't want her to be unfairly judged or scrutinized by anyone when she did recover and get released. We didn't want her to have to have some sort of stigma follow her around, and we wanted to protect her privacy as best we could. And allow her to share her journey with others if and when she was ready.

When B had her second break, it was difficult because we as a family began to come to terms with the fact that this may be a lifelong journey for her rather than an isolated episode. It proved that the first episode wasn't just a one-time hiccup. That this could potentially be a recurring issue. Which was a scary thought and a difficult concept to come to terms with. We had also just watched her come so far and make so much progress in her recovery, only for it to seem like that was all suddenly erased. After so many months of being flat from the medicine, she had finally been getting her energy back and it was seeming like the "old B" was finally returning. It was like she was just getting back to her old self, only for the rug to be pulled out from under us. I remember when we first realized that she was slipping into another episode and my heart breaking as I watched my mom sort of break down and say "she was just starting to come back to me." So, it was definitely a hard time for our family.

But at the same time, the second break was easier in some ways too. Easier because this time around we knew what to expect so it was a little easier navigating everything. And we at least had the prior experience of knowing that she could/would come out of the episode. The tone of the second episode was also a lot different than the first. This time she was manic and so rather than her being really scared and paranoid she was just very high energy and would say and do things that were, to be honest, sometimes very comical. So, there was a lot more levity and comic relief with the second episode. Not to say that we still weren't extremely concerned for her well-being and still going through a very hard time. But we were able to learn to laugh at some of the situations the second time around. For example, as B described earlier in the book - when she had us bringing all of those random bizarre items out to the car before heading to Lakeshore. We could not help but laugh at how ridiculous we probably looked carrying all those items out of the house into the van. We humored her and did it, but were just imagining what the neighbors must think, seeing all of us in an assembly line out of the house carrying things like a full-size organ, a globe and a statue of Mary and loading them into the van. Also, the moment where she proudly stated all of her self-appointed nicknames to the intake nurse at BryLin and then showed off her "Depends" disposable underwear and called herself Tommy Pickles. We were dying laughing. Or when she would point her "good vibes" stick (a twig that she'd found on the ground) and "zap" people with good vibes. We got a kick out of that too. When we were in the waiting room at Lakeshore she was pacing around the waiting room, kind of looking around the room suspiciously, and we could tell that she was sizing each person up to see if they needed good vibes. And we'd see her pause and kind of squint at a person who she clearly thought had bad vibes and we'd see her discreetly hold up the twig and point it in their direction. And we would just laugh and say "well, I guess that person needed good vibes." Or when she would gather random items and give little sermons on each item's meaning. At one point she had a pile of random household items collected on the table and was holding each one up, explaining to us the meaning behind it. She told us that some of the items represented people in her life. And she picked up a small pair of eyebrow tweezers out of the pile and told my mother that those tweezers represented her because she sometimes lovingly "picks" at her giving her constructive criticism and is her "kindest critic." Another thing we got a kick out of was when she didn't include my family's names on her initial visitor sheet at BryLin, but instead had the celebrities Ellen and Pink listed on there. We laughed a lot about that and just said, "Well I guess if we were going to get bumped off the list by someone at least it was some big celebrities." So again, as concerned and worried as we were, it did feel good to be able to find the levity and comic relief wherever we could.

The third episode didn't seem like as big of an event as the first two. Probably because one, she was able to stay home and two, it seemed to dissipate more quickly. Her being able to stay home and out of the hospital helped immensely. And by that point we at least had a better grasp on how to handle the situation and how to talk to and help B when she was feeling unstable. Not to say we weren't concerned, but again it did seem to get easier for us to handle it each time.

So, that first initial break was definitely the hardest. And my heart goes out to anyone going through it. Especially just because of the unknowns that come with it. As I said, it can be a terrifying feeling to not know if your loved one will come out of the episode. And then to just try to imagine what their future might look like and how their life might be irrevocably altered by this issue. If I were to give any advice to any family going through it, I would just say to try to hang in there, take it one day at a time, don't allow your mind to jump to the worst conclusions, advocate for your loved one and be involved. And don't be afraid to ask for meetings and to ask questions if you don't understand something. Also don't forget to take care of yourself in the midst of everything as well.

I know we've all tried to be there as allies for B in her recovery and to help however we can. She's said it's helped to just have us as a sounding board, to be able to ask us questions and kind of keep her mind in check if she's starting to have paranoid thoughts. But for the most part B has really taken the lead and responsibility in her recovery and we realize how lucky we are and how rare that can be in these situations. We marvel every day at her strength and her commitment to stability.

Reading through B's experiences in this book both broke my heart (because I can't imagine how scary and isolating it must have felt for her), but it was also fascinating in a lot of ways too. It was amazing to read the experience from her perspective instead of ours. Learning her reasoning behind the different behaviors and things she was saying, that seemed so strange and alarming to us at the time, gave me a whole new insight and deeper understanding into how her mind was working during those moments. And that in turn has made some of the mystery and "strangeness" of the behaviors a little less scary and more understandable now in hindsight. For example, the blanket over the head. To us, we were just seeing our loved one behaving in a very strange and alarming way. And sometimes it was really, really sad and heart wrenching to watch. But now since I've read exactly what was going through her mind during that moment, I understand it better. Or for example, in the book when she explained the meaning behind why she would put the lotion all over her body and in her hair, why she would rub tea bags on her skin, why she would wear certain eccentric clothing and underwear on her head, or why she so adamantly didn't want us drinking from the water pitcher at the hospital. These were all things that confused us so much at the time. So, it's fascinating and almost gratifying now to be able to read what her thought processes were in those moments. And gaining a better understanding of how her mind was working at the time has helped in understanding everything as a whole. And since it has helped in understanding what she was going through internally, hopefully that will be able to assist us in helping her in the future if she's ever in that mind space again.

This journey has also helped to give me more understanding and less judgement as a whole to anyone who is suffering from a mental health crisis. Even though maybe our first instinct might be to be afraid or even laugh at some of their behaviors and what they say, it's made me realize that it's better to approach the situation with compassion, and with the understanding that in their mind, there is deep meaning to what they're doing.

One thing I do wish people understood more, from a family member's perspective, is how hard it can be to get someone you love to seek help. Especially when they are in the middle of an episode. They aren't thinking clearly and coherently - they aren't capable of that. And so, trying to reason with them and point out logical things is near impossible. So, when people look to families to intervene and step in and "force" someone to seek help and treatment - it's not always that simple. Even in the midst of a mental health episode, a person does not lose their rights and autonomy. So, aside from a drastic measure, such as an involuntary hold at the hospital, they can't just be drugged and dragged and forced to go anywhere or do anything. I remember it also being difficult just in terms of trying to keep B safe without feeling like we were "holding her prisoner" so to speak, or infringing on her freedoms as an adult. For example, when she was at the height of her mania, she was displaying some unsafe behaviors like trying to play the bongos while driving or wanting to drive down to the Peace Bridge late at night. We had to restrict her access to the car in order to keep her safe and to prevent her from potentially harming others too. She was upset at the time about these restrictions, as she was not in the correct mindset to understand the reasoning and logic. So, to her, and to any outsider not privy to the situation, it might look like she was being unfairly treated or restricted. So again, it can be a difficult thing to balance between maintaining someone's autonomy and freedom while also trying to keep them safe. Only through persistence and patience and educating yourself can you truly learn to navigate these things successfully. And hopefully learn to communicate with your loved one effectively so that when it is necessary, you are able to convince them to seek treatment voluntarily. Or better yet, learn ways to intervene before it even gets to that point. It's not always foolproof or immediately successful. It's a commitment of constant learning and patience.

At the beginning of all of this, we were suddenly thrown into uncharted waters that we had no idea how to navigate. It was overwhelming to say the least. Like any family who has a loved one experiencing a health issue, we suddenly had a lot to juggle. Things like trying to research symptoms on our own to get some answers, navigating between all the different doctors and specialists, trying to find which hospital or treatment center would be the best fit for our loved one, which medications would be best or the least detrimental, the best course of action for a successful recovery, in addition to other logistics like health insurance, FMLA and job concerns. So again, we were juggling basically all the exhausting things that go along with a physical health issue - but added onto all of that was the stigma and shame that unfortunately often gets attached specifically to mental health issues. It can make seeking support and treatment that much more difficult. The experience has made me have a newfound sense of empathy, camaraderie and respect for anyone who has also had to navigate this complicated journey of mental health. In a way I could've never understood before. It's also made me appreciate just how underfunded this area of our healthcare system can be. How lacking resources can be. And I know that we are among the lucky ones. I know there are many who aren't so lucky. For whom such episodes end in tragedy, or who seem to remain in a constant cycle of episodes. A revolving door. It was heartbreaking to see some of the patients at the hospital who it was clear didn't really have any family or anyone to advocate for them or assist them in recovery. Many of them were such kind, sweet people who clearly just needed help. It made me that much more aware that those people deserve dignity and respect and proper care too.

I will say that we seem to have reached a stable period in this journey and for that I am so grateful. Reading this book brought back a lot of those painful memories when everything first happened, when we were so unsure whether or not we'd make it through or whether B would be okay. But reading it also made me feel so grateful too. Grateful that we did make it through, and to realize how far B has come. It made me marvel at her strength. At her perseverance and her steadfast commitment to her recovery and stability, which has been nothing short of amazing. It even allowed us to look back and laugh with her at a lot of the things that happened during the episodes, especially when she was manic. It created more of an openness around everything that happened, which I think has helped to take away some of the heaviness of it, and maybe helped to lessen some of the trauma surrounding it too.

As for that initial fear we all felt when everything first happened - the fear that the old B may never come back to us fully and that we might've lost the person we knew and loved forever - we needn't have worried. She is still the same loving, caring, hilarious, compassionate, brilliant and creative person that we've always known. Her pure, good heart never went anywhere, it was always there even during the depths of her episodes and during the hardest of times for her. She remains the same person she always was - only stronger and more resilient. I love her and am happy to say I am closer to her now more than ever. She's my big sister and remains one of the people I look up to and admire the most. She's made it through a more harrowing experience and she made it through with dignity and grace. And she came out of it with her good heart still intact. One of the great examples of that is that she wanted to help others by writing this book. I know I mentioned before about how there's often shame attached to mental illness. But in reality, it should be the exact opposite. People should be applauded and recognized for being able to navigate their way through it. And I just hope she knows how proud we all are of her and how she has handled her journey.

She named this section lifebuoys, saying that we are her life savers, and I hope she knows that she's ours too.

Being aware of the magnitude of how much my family dealt with during my episodes and how the situation made them feel, including during my periods of recovery, has given me the diligence and commitment to do my best to stay above water. It has given me even more motivation to take on the responsibility to do my best to make sure I don't experience another severe mental break. The last thing I want to do is put them through any more horrific and heart-wrenching situations if I am able to prevent it.

SILVER LINING

Cruising clouds collide with the moonlight
Relaxing summer nights by the firelight
As the clock starts to approach midnight
With another day putting up the good fight

As each cloud passes by
Find strength in your sorrow
Let your silver linings grow
With every tomorrow

Crystal clear sky brightened by the moonshine
Embers popping from the burning pine
Living for this moment in time
As I sit back and I unwind

As the stars glisten in the night sky
Focus on what makes you grateful
Positive and peaceful
Gaining thoughts that are stable

Cruising clouds collide with the moonlight
Followed by a crystal-clear sky brightened by the moonlight
With another day putting up the good fight
With thoughts that are stable, gaining insight

As each cloud passes by
And stars glisten in the night sky
Focus on what makes you grateful
And let your silver linings grow

-b. amber stark

Section VI
CALM WATERS

The past few years have been some of the most turbulent and challenging of my life, full of many highs and lows. But with certitude I can say I've finally reached a sense of peace and stability. I've been fortunate to have been able to navigate my journey so far, and for now the waters seem to have calmed. Along the way I've gained many tools and strategies that have helped me. And in this section, I hope to be able to provide some guidance and advice that might help someone in the midst of their own storm. When I first started this journey, I remember seeking out resources and advice from books, documentaries, and experiences of those who had been through it. And now I hope to be that for someone else.

I used to get caught up in the stigma of mental health disorders. Sometimes half the battle of dealing with mental health issues is dealing with the stigma that comes with it. It can feel debilitating at times and be hard to overcome the fear of judgment from others. This fear of judgment gets in the way and makes it harder for individuals to gain acceptance of issues they may be experiencing and to further seek treatment. Initially, when I was presented with the fact that I have a mental disorder, the first thing that crossed my mind above anything else was what other people were going to think of me. Due to stigma, I was immediately under the impression I would no longer be accepted and developed a sense of denial regarding the whole diagnosis. I came to realize once I shifted my mindset into accepting the diagnosis, I was in a better position to receive the treatment I needed. This has allowed me to mend and essentially grow into a more grounded person. And I continue to fight to be a better me each day to prove to people that I am not any different than them.

To anyone that may be given a mental health classification, I know it is a heavy weight to hear such words. But know that there are so many other people out there that have been in similar situations as you. And that a classification is just a way to pinpoint what's going on so you are able to receive the best treatment and live a fulfilling life. It is not anything to be ashamed of and it's not something that defines you. I recently came across the quote, "There is strength in the surrender" by K. Tolnoe. I reflected on the meaning of this quote and how it related to me. It's as if once I surrendered to the fact that I have mental health issues, I was able to gain the strength and resolve to manage it. Accepting it has allowed me to focus on what I need to do, resulting in the ability for me to lead a fulfilling life. It is like I have been able to free myself from being a prisoner of my own mind, and free myself from being shackled by the stigma or shame of a diagnosis.

I think it's important to help people understand more about what goes on with mental health issues. It's part of the reason that I wrote this book. Hopefully gaining a better understanding will help with eliminating the stigma in society. I want others to understand that when an individual is going through a mental break, they may find deep meaning in things that they think and the things that they do. To my family and others at the hospital, I probably looked like a lunatic. Like a crazy person pacing around with a blanket over my head. It was probably a bizarre sight. To the outside world the things I would say and do probably seemed strange, unnerving, scary, even at times comical. But to me, it made perfect sense. I always try to keep this in mind, and I wish others would too, when seeing someone acting strange. I try to gain a better understanding of what the person may be thinking or feeling that would cause them to act in such a way. I try to remember that even though to someone of sound mind the behaviors may seem peculiar, they probably seem rational and have deep meaning to the person displaying the behavior. In these situations, I try to be compassionate rather than being judgmental. Just as I wouldn't judge someone for having side effects from diseases like cancer or leukemia, I don't judge someone who is suffering from mental health issues. Because it is just as much out of their control as any of those physical health issues I mentioned.

Leaving mental health issues unchecked is where problems arise. I know that coming to terms with the fact that you may need help is not always easy. And I also realize that trying to figure out what it is you need to do to help yourself is a lot easier said than done. But even if all you can manage is to let someone know how you're feeling and ask them for help, it's a good place to start. I know it's possible for some people to find it difficult to find someone they trust to turn to. But please know that there are always resources and help available to you. Even if you don't feel you have a close family member or friend, there are confidential hotlines and other services that can be lifelines for you. And I've included some at the end of this book. With that being said, in the end it's up to the individual to make the change to better themselves. Sure, others can help you and I am sure they are more than happy to. But they cannot make the change for you. It is mainly up to you. And it can be done. You have to have faith in yourself. If anything, start small and over time your progress will build up and be worth it in the end. Take one day at a time and try your best to fight to be better to allow yourself to live a fulfilling life. Nobody deserves to live in misery, and the thing is you don't have to.

For those people that are worried about a loved one, don't be afraid to ask them about it or to step in to get them help. With that being said I know that confronting someone with the fact that they need help is not always an easy task. There can be the fear of a potentially bad reaction from them - especially from someone that might not be in the right mindset. I personally have been on both sides. I've been the one who needed to be confronted and I've also been the one who needed to confront a loved one who I was concerned about. And I struggled with approaching them because I worried about how they would react – but I finally reached a point where I knew it was something that needed to be done. Something we could not let go on any longer. And as far as being on the other side of it, having my family sit me down and convince me to get help was the best thing to happen to me. It was the first step to me living a better life. In the end it ended up being exactly what was needed for me. Having those difficult conversations is necessary. And I know how difficult it can be to try to assist someone in getting the help they need because it ultimately comes down to the individual. You can't necessarily force someone to want the change in some cases. All you can do is continue to support them, letting them know you're there. As an outsider, sometimes it is easier to be aware of factors that may be making situations worse or harder to overcome. Continue having conversations and kindly remind them of those things that you think make their situation worse or things that you think can make it better. Offer them the time to speak about what is on their mind and listen. Sometimes just listening can be helpful. If you find it hard to communicate your concerns through conversation, another option is to write a letter and read it to them, as my family did for me. And for those of you that have tried to help someone that may not seem responsive to the help, know that you are doing your best and all you can do is continue to provide your support.

The support of family and friends is so important – but it also cannot replace the invaluable resource of a licensed professional. I realize that for many people, seeking out the help of a psychiatrist or counselor can be an intimidating and daunting step. But it is an important step that is worth it. They are knowledgeable and can provide unbiased professional advice as well as strategies, techniques and tools that will be useful in times of need. Furthermore, I'm not one for pill-pushing but sometimes medication is necessary in order to get to where you want to be. Being on medication can be tough, but work with your psychiatrist to manage it to a point where you are able to lead a functional and fulfilling life. When I was apprehensive about taking medication, my psychiatrist explained things to me using an analogy. He explained that people with Diabetes need to take insulin to be functional and survive. So, I had to look at my situation in a similar way. I had to look at it from the perspective that the medication might just be something I would need in order to be functional, much like a Diabetic with insulin. I got to a point where I wanted to get things under control for good. And I figured that the sooner I was able to get things under control, the sooner I would be able to be the person I wanted to be and to live the life I wanted to live. I finally accepted that medication may be the best way to do that in assisting me in overcoming my issues. Before this conversation with the doctor, I had always focused on getting off the medication completely as my main goal simply because I did not want to be on it. But I shifted the focus of my main goal to wanting to get better and reach a point of maintaining mental stability. After giving the medicine a chance and being on a low dose long term, I have found that I am functional again. My thoughts are more controlled and I am able to do things I want and be the person I want to be without drowning in my own thoughts. I realized it didn't have to be "all or nothing" with medication. I didn't have to choose between two extremes of either being a non-functional highly medicated flat person or a completely unmedicated manic paranoid person. I could find a balance between the two that worked for me. Where I can be on the right dose to keep my mind in check, while also still allowing myself to feel alive and engaged in life. I didn't need to always have the ultimate goal of getting off medication completely, I just needed to find the right balance.

A quote I once read by Andy Andrews states, "Discipline is the ability to do something you don't want to do, in order to get a result, you really want to get." This can be applied to many aspects of life. For me, I have become disciplined about taking medication and also about not consuming alcohol. When it comes to alcohol, I would always regret how horrible I would feel in the days following a night of drinking, and to me it is not worth it. I started to focus on the idea that alcohol is a short-term pleasure. And avoiding short-term pleasures, such as alcohol, can be hard because of the instant gratification. In some situations, alcohol is used to mask issues when someone is struggling, but ends up just making life harder to handle in the end. After thinking about it, I asked myself the questions: Would you rather sacrifice a good life for a short-term pleasure? Or sacrifice a short-term pleasure for a good life? Subsequently, I began to reflect on the idea of long-term pleasures and how they can be more rewarding and fulfilling than short-term pleasures. And, for me, I considered gaining control of my thoughts and maintaining my stability as a long-term pleasure. The idea of living a fulfilling life was more rewarding to me. So, I needed to work toward making a change for the better. Life-changes can be tough and can take time. And if we don't usually see the change right away, it can make it harder to stick to working toward the change. But the key is to be patient and to discipline yourself. Consuming alcohol makes my mind weak and makes it difficult to handle stressful situations or disturbing thoughts. I have found that becoming disciplined when it comes to not consuming alcohol allows for more clarity. And I think having more clarity makes it easier to manage turbulent thoughts and situations. And in the end, having clarity and maintaining a stable mind is more rewarding and allows me to lead a more fulfilling life. Overall, I feel I am a happier person from becoming disciplined when it comes to taking medication and not consuming alcohol.

For those of you in a dark place, focus on the silver linings. If you're struggling to identify your silver linings, try to think about things that make you grateful and happy. Anything. That is how I started. Even if it's something as simple as something you like to eat, something you like to watch on T.V., a song you like to listen to or sing, or someone you like to be with - take that and incorporate that into your life more. Try not to focus on the negative situations - that just brings you down and floods your mind with negative energy. Focus on what you CAN do. Focus on the positive with every experience and situation you are met with - I believe there is always good in every situation. Or at least a lesson to learn that will lead to growth and strength. But you won't see it if you don't actively direct your mind toward it. I personally like the following quote from the movie *Silver Linings Playbook.* In the movie, the character that suffers from Bipolar Disorder states, "I'm gonna take all this negativity and I'm gonna use it as fuel and I'm gonna find a silver lining." This statement is powerful. Using the negative energy to your advantage to get to a better place is a good tactic to practice. And I think once you start identifying silver linings, you start to realize more things you are grateful for over time which contributes to a healthier, happier mindset. You need to train your mind to think in a more positive manner. The more you think positive the easier it becomes

- almost like second nature. As a result, you become lighter and it's easier to navigate through life.

I also think routine is important. One routine that I try to stick to that I think is prominent in maintaining stability is following a proper sleep schedule. It sounds simple, but being well rested really makes all the difference for me in being able to maintain a healthy mind. Lack of sleep and fatigue can trigger stress which can often lead to symptoms. I think it is not only important to make sure you are getting enough sleep, but also that you're on a consistent sleep schedule around the same time each day. This gets your body accustomed to a sleep cycle and helps keep your mind balanced. Another seemingly simple but effective practice that helps me, especially on hard days, is taking a hot shower. It's almost therapeutic for me. Sometimes when you're in a low place and finding it hard to even get out of bed, if you can muster up enough energy to get up and at least take a hot shower, it can make all the difference. It can be that first small step toward making you feel better. Additionally, developing healthy, positive outlets such as writing, yoga, exercise, music, crafts, and cooking can help you through life's obstacles.

Another essential element of maintaining stability is to learn to identify your triggers and early warning signs that occur as an episode is approaching. Pinpointing triggers can help you avoid them and prevent the onset of symptoms. Being able to identify subtle signs leading up to an episode can allow for immediate treatment and overall quicker recovery. Two triggers for me that I believe contribute to the onset of having issues include lack of sleep and poor management of stress. And the subtlest signs of paranoia alert me and I am sure to try and talk myself through these thoughts and avoid feeding into them.

For those struggling, talking about your situation or writing about it can be what saves you. I will say that writing about my experiences and feelings was great therapy for me. Even as I'm writing this now and with spending the last four years recapping my journey, it's as if I have a sense of closure with this chapter in my life. The memories do not seem to weigh me down as much. I even seldomly think about my experiences anymore.

Since writing about my experiences, it is as if I became detached from the memories emotionally. And if I do think about them, it is not as heavy of a weight. Writing about what I have been through has been a therapy that has created a foundation to a new way of life for me. Speaking to people, whether it be family members or professionals, has created an outlet that prevents me from falling deep under the irrational thoughts and feelings I experience. Sometimes when you're not in a good mind space it can be difficult and overwhelming to try to navigate through your thoughts. And the more you bottle up the thoughts the harder it becomes to deal with them. So, opening up and talking to someone about disturbing thoughts that may be weighing you down can give you an opportunity to release the negative emotions attached to the thoughts.

I also think it's important to become educated on mental disorders and how they affect the general population. Diseases of the brain are scary because they can't be seen, they aren't a tangible thing. And a diagnosis and course of treatment aren't always straightforward and easy to find. With physical injuries, you can look at blood tests and x-rays and a lot of times receive a pretty concrete diagnosis and prognosis. When it is your brain and your mind that seem to be broken, those issues are a lot more complex to explain, to understand, and to treat.

As far as what may have caused this new reality and new way of life for me? I think it's possible I always had a predisposition to develop a mental health disorder. I also think that the way I managed my emotions and stress throughout my life and the use of drugs and alcohol contributed to the onset and development of the condition. So, I believe it was a mix of both nature and nurture. I believe the condition would have developed, no matter what, over time. But it is possible that my drug use and inability to manage stress well triggered the onset and acted as a catalyst to me developing the condition. Regardless, I am here now and my recovery and maintenance continue each day. I still consider myself in my third stretch of recovery. And I am proud to say that I haven't had a major episode since the Summer of 2016.

As for now, I'm happy to say that I don't walk around covered by a blanket that I think has protective properties, I don't wear underwear on my head, and I do not think my family members are clones. But I do still have my peacock sneakers. And some of my best days are spent walking around in my peacock sneakers. A side note, I still think honey is liquid gold and it's delicious.

I do believe we all go a little mad sometimes. But like my mother said to me growing up, take control of your emotions. Take control of your mind. Don't let emotions control you. Aside from that, you need to be honest with yourself. Seek help. Be honest with your help. And be your best advocate. Listen to your doctor. If you don't agree with something, then discuss it and share your opinion. Only you know how you truly feel inside. Communicate this with your psychiatrist and counselor. Follow the schedule given for medicine and stay the course. And stay clean. These points embody the best recipe for a successful recovery. Commitment to these points also enables a better chance at lowering the dosage of medication. Higher doses can have negative side effects as I have mentioned, such as a flat affect or weight gain. If you need to be prescribed a high dose - know that it does not need to be long term and can be temporary. But be mindful that medicine is just a crutch to get you in a position to take control. Medicine cannot do all the work. Keep in mind you have to try your best to do your part too. Some days are going to be easier than others. Embrace the easy ones and stay strong on the harder days. Life's a challenge. No matter what, everyone has their own battles. Don't give up the fight. Some advice I was given following my second episode was, "Every breakdown has the potential to be a breakthrough." This advice has motivated me in a way that I was eager to continue to fight for mental stability each day until I reached a breakthrough from what I had experienced. I continue to fight to maintain that stability every day.

Needless to say, the mind can play tricks sometimes and make you feel like life's not worth it. Throughout this journey, I've had days where I felt so low, I've had days where I felt so flat and like a nobody, days where I struggled to get out of bed and felt like I couldn't go on. But I fought through them, kept going, and that has allowed me to have some of my best days. Days where I feel so happy and lucky that I get to be here, to be alive and to be able to spend them with the people I love the most. So, if you're reading this and you're like me in any way, have struggled with mental health or have faced any personal struggle at all, I'm here to tell you and to remind you that the fight is worth it. It will always be worth it and it's possible to come out on the other side a stronger and better, more complete person. And know that you're never alone and that there are always people out there who have gone through what you have and can relate and help you. Whenever I am struggling, I try to focus on things I am grateful for in my life. I focus on silver linings in my life to help pull me out of the darkness. I often recite the mantra "Today is going to be a good day." I especially say this on the mornings I wake up and don't feel like doing life. I will even say it and repeat it out loud several times. I have also found that on the tough mornings, if I splash cold water on my face it helps to jump-start my day and help me snap out of it. I know doing these things sounds silly. But I have found that the little things make a big difference. I have learned to persevere, especially on the bad days. Keep a positive mind no matter what. View the glass as half full. And as my father would tell me: everything in moderation. It's all about balance. That's the best way to improve and live a better life.

Will I have another episode in the future? I do not know. Only time will tell. But I will say I am diligent and work hard to try not to. I strive to continue to grow each day to be a better me. And not just for me but for the people around me. And I think there is always work that can be done. Nobody is perfect. I've learned to exorcise my demons using positive, healthy outlets such as writing, music, dance, exercise, yoga, bike riding, walking, crafts, coloring, and communicating with my supports. Every once in a while, negative energy will try to creep in, but I'm always sure to turn to my positive outlets. Communicating with those I trust most is an important tool for me. When I am paranoid, I ask them questions and they reassure me that everything is alright. When the negative energy seeps in, I've learned to talk myself through it and "put the glass down" at the end of the day. This phrase came from a video I saw on social media. In the video a professor takes a full glass of water and asks his students how heavy the glass is. The professor goes on to explain that if you hold the glass of water for a short time, it is not as heavy of a weight. But the longer you hold on to the glass, the heavier it becomes. And after a while it will even start to hurt your arm. Therefore, you should "put the glass down" and erase any worry or stress you have at the end of each day. If you don't, it will snowball and be worse than it needs to be. I keep this analogy in mind as my days go on and it helps prevent me from becoming overwhelmed with negative thoughts, helps me navigate the sometimes choppy, sometimes calm waters of my mind, and helps prevent the tidal waves from rolling in.

"I'll stand up to your tidal waves
   Fighting through the helpless and all alone
   I'll stand up to your tidal waves
   Fighting to keep my mind in a healthy zone

   I'll stand up to your tidal waves
   Fighting through the unexpected pain
   I'll stand up to your tidal waves
   Fighting to keep my mind sane"
 -b. amber stark

BREAKTHROUGH

When the weight is upon your shoulders
As if you're carrying a ton of boulders

You just need to keep your head up
And break through those bricks

Even when you think the tunnel is closed
There is a light on the other side you need to expose

You just need to keep your head up
And break through those bricks

Keep up the fight and the light will filter through
The bricks will fall and you'll reach a breakthrough

You just need to keep your head up
And break through those bricks
-b. amber stark

RESOURCES

Recommended Books that have personally helped me in my journey:

- *The Untethered Soul* By Michael A. Singer
- *The Voice of Knowledge* By Don Miguel Ruiz
- *The Four Agreements* By Don Miguel Ruiz
- *The Fifth Agreement* By Don Miguel Ruiz and Don Jose Ruiz
- *The Mastery of Self* By Don Miguel Ruiz Jr.
- *The Mastery of Life* By Don Miguel Ruiz Jr.
- *The Circle of Fire* By Don Miguel Ruiz

Recommended Documentary:

- *Stutz*, Directed by: Jonah Hill

Mental Health Resources:

- Suicide and Crisis Lifeline: 988 -call or text 988
- Crisis text line: text HOME to 741-741
- NAMI (National Alliance on Mental Illness): www.nami.org -this website provides a Helpline Resource Directory database with a wide variety of support options (top right drop down menu select Get Help select NAMI Resource Directory)
- NAMI Helpline: 800-950-6264 or text "Helpline" to 62640 (available M-F 10am-10pm ET)
- NIMH (National Institute of Mental Health) www.nimh.nih.gov -provides information regarding mental disorders and related topics
- FindTreatment.gov -provides help for substance use disorders, addiction and mental illness
- American Psychiatric Association Foundation -find a psychiatrist
- American Academy of Child and Adolescent Psychiatry -find psychiatrist for children and adolescents

- American Psychological Association -find a psychologist

- www.PsychU.org -resources for mental health for: self, loved one, health care professionals

MENTAL HEALTH RESOURCES AND SERVICES (BUFFALO, NY):

- 211wny.org

- BestSelf Behavioral Health (716) 884-0888
  -All BestSelf clinics offer walk-ins and same day appointments

- Al-Anon (716) 856-2520

- BryLin Hospital – Mental Health. Services

- 1263 Delaware Ave. Buffalo, NY 14209
  (716) 886-8200

- Behavioral Healthcare Network -website

- Buffalo Psychiatric Center Office of Mental Health -website

- Child and Family Services
  330 Delaware Ave. Buffalo, NY 14202
  (716) 842-2750

- CMH Counseling
  153 W Utica St. Buffalo, NY 14222
  (716) 884-7569

- Core Mental Health Counseling
  737 Delaware Ave. Buffalo, NY 14202
  (716) 247-6425

- CPH Mental Health Counseling
  737 Delaware Ave. Suite 216, Buffalo, NY 14209
  (716) 322-6349

- Crisis Services
  100 River Rock Dr. Suite 300, Buffalo, NY 14207
  (716) 834-3131

- ECMC Health Services
  462 Grider St. Buffalo, NY 14215
  Endeavor Health Services

- 526 Walden Ave. #400,
  Cheektowaga, NY 14225
  (716) 895-6700

- Family Counseling Associates
  884 Brighton Rd. Tonawanda, NY 14150

- Gateway Longview – Behavioral Health Clinic, Symphony Circle
  10 Symphony Circle Buffalo, NY 14201
  (716) 783-3100

- Greater Buffalo Counseling Center
  410 Minnesota Ave. Buffalo, NY 14214
  (716) 833-5993

- Horizon Health Services
  (716) 831-1800

- Main Stay Counseling
  2178 Main St. Buffalo, NY 14214
  (716) 704-8268

- Mental Health – Erie County
  95 Franklin St. Buffalo, NY 14202

- Mental Health Advocates of WNY
  1021 Broadway 5th floor Buffalo, NY 14212
  (716) 886-1242
- NAMI: National Alliance on Mental Illness Buffalo and Erie County
  (716) 226-6264

- Narins Eating Disorder Center
  2430 North Forest Road Amherst, NY 14068
  (716) 688-5372

- Spectrum Health and Human Services
  (716) 710-5172

- Substance Abuse and Mental Health Services Administration -website

- Transitional Services Inc
  389 Elmwood Ave. Buffalo, NY 14222

- WNY Psychotherapy Services -website

Rehab Facilities:

- Harbor of Grace
  PO Box 872
  437 Girard St. Havre De Grace, MD 21078
  (443) 502-8606

- Futures Recovery Healthcare
  701 Old Dixie Hwy Tequesta, FL 33469
  (866) 327-3183

- Sunshine Behavioral Health Facilities:
  855-972-7239
  www.sunshinebehavioralhealth.com

- Chapters Capistrano
  1525 Buena Vista, San Clemens, CA 92672

- Monarch Shores
  27123 Calle Arroyo #2121, San Juan Capistrano, CA 92675

- Mountain Springs
  1865 Woodmoor Dr, Monument, CO 80132

- Willow Springs Recovery
  1128 TX-21, Bastrop, TX 78602

- Lincoln Recovery
  19067 W Frontage Rd, Raymond, IL 62569-505

www.ingramcontent.com/pod-product-compliance
Lightning Source LLC
Chambersburg PA
CBHW030109300326
41934CB00033B/327